Parents' Journey with Child's Mental Health

Bruce M. Gonzalez

TABLE OF CONTENTS

LIST OF TABLES

ABSTRACT

The impacts of stigma on people with lived-experience are widely recognized, however, stigma has been noted to extend to family members. The current investigation examines how specific types of stigma experienced by parents/caregivers (N=250) of children with mental health challenges are related to symptoms of depression and attitudes towards help-seeking. Results found that higher levels of public stigma, self-stigma, and vicarious stigma were associated with higher levels of depression and were differentially associated with attitudes towards help-seeking. Findings from this investigation add to the small body of literature examining stigma experienced by parents/caregivers of children with mental health challenges.

CHAPTER 1

INTRODUCTION

According to the Child and Adolescent Health Measurement Initiative, 2019 National Survey of Children's Health, an average of 22.1% of children (ages 3-17) across the United States have at least one mental, emotional, developmental, or behavioral problem. For children, mental health and related challenges can have negative impacts on various domains of life such as physical health, family relationships, school/academic performance, and social support (Patel, Flisher, Hetrick, & McGorry, 2007). Raising a child with mental health challenges can be an extremely difficult task for parents/caregivers, and the experiences of stigma further compound these challenges.

Stigma has been defined as a "mark" or an "undesirable characteristic" (e.g., having mental health challenges), which results in prejudice and discrimination towards an individual (Goffman, 1963). The effects of stigma on people with lived-experience (e.g., a person with mental health challenges) are widely recognized in the research; this applies equally to adults as well as children with mental health challenges. However, stigma has also been found to cast a wide net, extending to others such as family members of the person with lived-experience (e.g., the parents/caregivers of a child with mental health challenges) (Corrigan & Miller, 2004; Corrigan, Watson, & Miller, 2006; Moses, 2014; Perlick et al., 2011; Robinson & Brewster, 2016). For example, a neighbor endorsing public stigma may report, *"That parent should be ashamed of themselves for causing their child's mental health challenges."* Research on the effects of stigma has mainly focused on the children with mental health challenges, giving little attention to their parents/caregivers (Eaton, Ohan, Stritzke & Corrigan, 2016; Gottman, Katz, & Hooven, 1996; McKeague,

Hennessy, O'Driscoll-Lawrie, & Heary, 2022; Moses, 2014). Thus, there is a lack of knowledge regarding the stigma experiences of parents/caregivers of children with mental health challenges.

Parents/caregivers of children with mental health challenges have been found to endorse aspects of self-stigma, specifically regarding public stereotypes of blame and feelings of incompetence (Corrigan & Wassel, 2008; Eaton et al., 2016; Moses, 2014; Perlick et al., 2011). For example, a parent may think, *"I am a bad parent because my child has mental health challenges."* These experiences of public and self-stigma may lead to issues with help-seeking and symptoms of depression (Corrigan, Druss, & Perlick, 2014; Eaton et al., 2020). In other words, parents/caregivers may not seek out services for their child in order to avoid stigma. Vicarious stigma is a fairly new and additional area of research, which describes the emotional response a parent/caregiver may experience when witnessing their child with mental health challenges being stigmatized by others in the context of this investigation (Corrigan & Miller, 2004; Serchuk, Corrigan, Reed, & Ohan, 2021). Vicarious stigma experienced by parents/caregivers may have a similar, negative impact on help-seeking and depression. However, it is possible that vicarious stigma has an energizing effect on parents, which may create motivation to engage in help-seeking.

The present paper examines outcomes related to different types of stigmas experienced by parents/caregivers of children with mental health challenges. The proposed model examines the path from public stigma towards parents/caregivers of children with mental health challenges, to self-stigma, to diminished help-seeking and increased symptoms of depression. The model also examines a separate pathway from public stigma towards people with mental health challenges, to vicarious stigma, to positive attitudes towards help-seeking for their child and increased symptoms of depression. Overall the model examines the relationships between public stigmas, self-stigma, vicarious stigma, depression, and help-seeking attitudes within a population of parents/caregivers of children with mental health challenges (Figure 1).

Figure 1

Hypothesized Model

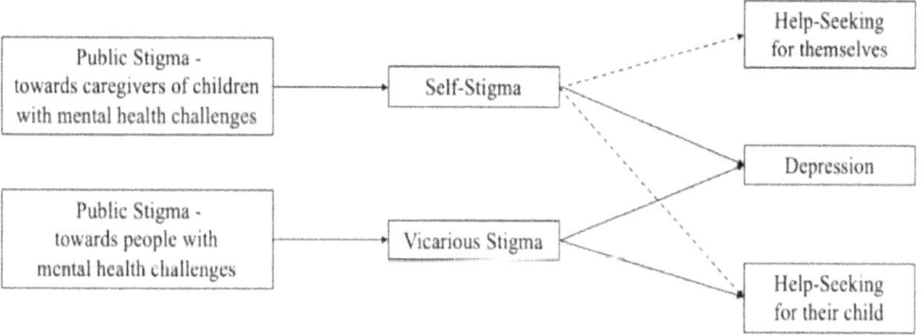

Note. Dashed line indicates negative relationship

This dissertation will begin by defining and reviewing specific forms of stigmas that parents/caregivers of children with mental health challenges face – focusing on public stigma, self-stigma, and vicarious stigma. Second, the impacts of stigma related to symptoms of depression and help-seeking attitudes for parents/caregivers of children with mental health challenges will be discussed. A summary of the proposed hypotheses is provided, which is followed by the methods for the current investigation. The findings and results will then be presented. Finally, a discussion section summarizing the findings, strengths and weaknesses of the study, and future directions will conclude this manuscript.

CHAPTER 2

LITERATURE REVIEW

The first part of this section will begin by reviewing the social-cognitive model of stigma, a useful framework for understanding the process of stigma. A description of the social-cognitive model will first be presented in terms of adults with mental health challenges, for which the model was developed, and then children with mental health challenges. Then extending the social-cognitive model to parents of children with mental health challenges, who are a special case called associative sigma will be discussed. In each case, there will be description of the impact of stigma on each group: adults with mental health challenges, children with mental health challenges, and parents of children with mental health challenges. The chapter then provides introduction and consideration of vicarious stigma, a fairly new concept of stigma that extends from the person with lived experience to family members.

2.1   On the Stigma of Mental Illness

The social-cognitive model of stigma is a framework with three components – stereotypes, prejudice, and discrimination (Corrigan, 2000; Corrigan & Watson, 2002), see Figure 2. Stereotypes are generalizations regarding the characteristics, attributes, and behaviors identified by others regarding members of a group (Corrigan & Watson, 2002; Hilton & Von Hipple, 1996; Judd & Park, 1993). An example of a common stereotype regarding adults with mental health challenges is that they are dangerous (Corrigan, 2000; Corrigan et al., 2003; Link et al., 1999; Parcesepe & Cabassa, 2013; Pescosolido et al., 2007; Pescosolido et al., 2008; Steadman, 1981). It is important to note that awareness of a given stereotype does not indicate agreement (Jussim, Manis, Nelson, & Soffin, 1995).

For instance, having knowledge of the stereotype from the example above does not imply that the reader agrees with the stereotype. Individuals who endorse stereotypes and experience a negative emotional response are exhibiting prejudice (Corrigan & Watson, 2002; Devine, 1989, 1995; Hilton & Von Hipple, 1996). For example, a person would be prejudiced against adults with mental health challenges if they agree with the dangerousness stereotype, and, in turn, feel scared of people with mental health challenges. Discrimination is then the behavioral reaction to prejudice (Corrigan & Watson, 2002). For instance, an individual may discriminate against people with mental health challenges by avoiding them, in response to their fear of dangerousness (Corrigan & Matthews, 2003).

Figure 2

The Social Cognitive Model of Stigma, Including Public Stigma and Self-Stigma

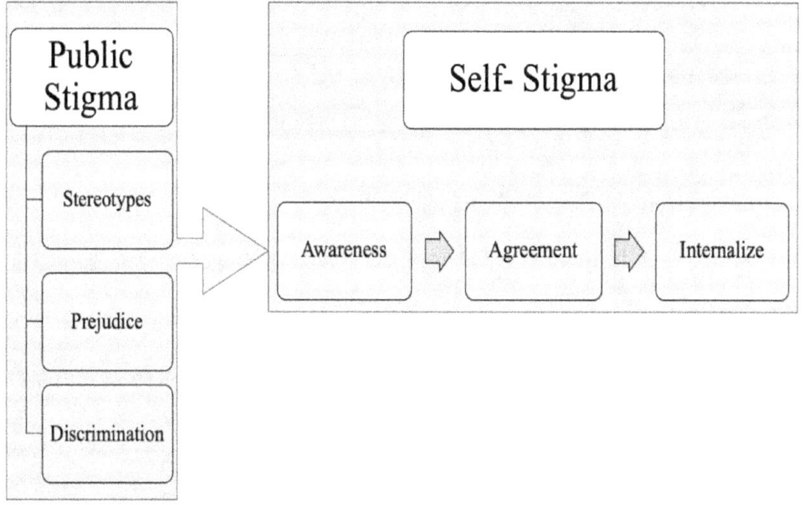

Public stigma is defined as when members of the public endorse stereotypes, prejudice, and discrimination towards an adult with mental health challenges (Corrigan,

Watson, & Miller, 2006; Goffman, 1963; Phelan, Bromet, & Link, 1998; Robinson & Brewster, 2016; Shi et al., 2019). In a systematic review on public stigma of mental illness in the United States, Parcesepe and Cabassa (2013) found that adults with mental illness faced public stigma related to dangerousness, blame, and incompetence. Experiences of public stigma can be viewed as a loss of opportunity. For instance, adults with mental illness experiencing public stigma may face discrimination in the form of exclusion from social/family gatherings, or they may be rejected for employment or housing (Parcesepe & Cabassa, 2013). For example, a potential landlord may think, "*Allowing that person with mental illness to move into my building seems dangerous* (stereotypes), *I worry about the safety of the other tenants* (prejudice). *I am not going to approve their application* (discrimination)." Potential consequences to disclosing mental health challenges may include blame, disapproval, and avoidance by others (Corrigan & Matthews, 2003). Deciding whether to disclose mental health challenges or conceal them can be an extremely difficult decision to make for individuals (Homes & River, 1998; Corrigan & Matthews, 2003). These experiences of public stigma can impact adults with mental health challenges in different ways.

2.1.1   On the Impacts of Public Stigma. Individual responses to public stigma can vary. Many individuals internalize the experience of public stigma and suffer negative consequences. Self-stigma is defined as the process of becoming aware of, agreeing with, and internalizing public stereotypes (Corrigan & Watson, 2002; see Figure 2). Literature examining adults with mental health challenges has demonstrated a link between experiences of self-stigma and negative emotional experiences such as diminished feelings of self-esteem and self-efficacy as well as poor health outcomes (Corrigan &

Rao, 2012; Corrigan, Watson, & Barr, 2006; Drapalski et al., 2013; Watson et al., 2007). For example, an adult experiencing self-stigma may think, *"I am so incompetent because of how I let my mental health challenges get in the way of my job performance* (stereotypes and prejudice)*! I am too ashamed to show my face at the holiday party tonight* (discrimination)*."* Research has also shown that higher levels of perceived public stigma associated with mental health challenges is related to higher levels of the self-stigma, which is related to more negative attitudes towards seeking help for problems related to mental health challenges (Vogal, Wade, & Ascheman, 2009; Vogel, Wade, & Hackler, 2007). Overall, experiences of self-stigma have the potential to affect adults in various negative ways.

As mentioned above, deciding whether to disclose mental health challenges or to conceal them can be an extremely difficult, and not an "all-or-nothing" type of decision (Homes & River, 1998; Corrigan & Matthews, 2003; Corrigan & Rao, 2012). Adults may engage in social avoidance, or self-imposed discrimination, to avoid the experiences of stigma by completely avoiding others (Corrigan & Rao, 2012). Secrecy coping is another method, in which adults decide to avoid experiences of stigma by concealing mental health challenges (Link et al., 1997). Adults who perceive higher levels of self-stigma are more likely to endorse secrecy coping (Corrigan & Matthews, 2003; Luoma et al., 2007). In other words, adults with mental health challenges who are experiencing high levels of self-stigma are more likely to opt for concealment over disclosure. Although there are potential negative consequences, disclosure of mental health challenges has the capability of reducing negative impacts of perceived stigma (Corrigan et al., 2010).

When opting for disclosure, strategies in which adults with mental health challenges may engage range from selective disclosure, to indiscriminate disclosure, to broadcasting (Corrigan & Rao, 2012). Potential benefits to disclosure can include reducing stigma-related distress as well as facilitate support for the individual with mental health challenges (Corrigan et al., 2010; Corrigan & Rao, 2012). Contact with others who have lived experience (e.g., other adults with mental health challenges) and education have been identified as having positive effects on reducing the effects of stigma (Corrigan et al., 2012). For example, an adult who is willing to disclose may have more opportunities to meet other people with lived experience. Having open conversations about their lived experience with others, this person may be invited to attend a support group with other individuals and/or is able to find appropriate referrals for services. Hearing and learning from other adults' experiences has the potential to reduce the self-stigmatizing attitudes of blame and incompetence the individual may be endorsing as well.

The social-cognitive model of stigma is useful for examining the stigma experiences of adults with mental health challenges. Both public stigma and self-stigma can have far reaching, negative impacts on targeted individuals. In summary, these stigma experiences can lead to losses of opportunities (e.g., social support, employment) as well as negative emotional (e.g., low self-efficacy), behavioral (e.g., less willingness to disclose or seek help), and health consequences. Although opting for disclosure may potentially reduce negative consequences of stigma, it is important for individuals to weigh the potential positive and negative consequences of doing so.

2.2   Stigma Experienced by Children with Mental Health Challenges

Similar to the experiences of adults, children and adolescence are also stigmatized for their mental health challenges. Adults (e.g., family members, neighbors, teachers, doctors) are not the only perpetrators of public stigma towards children with mental health challenges. Stigma is prevalent across developmental stages and can start at a young age (Corrigan & Watson, 2007; Ferrie, Miller, & Hunter, 2020; Heary, Hennessy, Swords, & Corrigan, 2017; O'Driscoll et al., 2012). The public seems to have similar stigmatizing beliefs about children with mental health challenges, endorsing beliefs regarding dangerousness, blame, shame, and criminality (Parcesepe & Cabassa, 2013). For instance, utilizing the social-cognitive model of stigma, other children who endorse the dangerousness stereotype may feel scared of their peer with mental health challenges (i.e., prejudice), which can result in excluding the child from social situations such as birthday parties (i.e. discrimination). Another example can include a teacher endorsing common stereotypes and prejudice of blame and incompetence, and, in turn, overlooking (i.e. discrimination) the student experiencing mental health challenges. It can be common for children with mental health challenges to experience discrimination in the form of bullying by their peers (Moses, 2010). Peers who endorse stereotypes and attitudes of blame and shame may engage in various forms of bullying directed towards a child with mental health challenges (e.g., making mean "jokes," physically hurting the child, getting the child into trouble/manipulation).

2.2.1   On the Impacts of Public Stigma on Children. Children may respond to public forms of stigma in a variety of ways, which can include the process of becoming aware of, agreeing with, and internalizing public attitudes as their own. Children with mental health challenges have been found to endorse self-stigmatizing beliefs, and many such beliefs are similar to adults. Children have been found to endorse stereotypes/prejudice of shame, embarrassment, blame, feeling "weak," and feeling "different"/ "not normal" (Ferrie, Miller, & Hunter, 2020; Hanlon & Swords, 2019; Keyes, Nolte, & Williams, 2018; Mitten et al., 2016; Moses, 2015). In a mixed-methods systematic review examining psychosocial outcomes of mental illness stigma in children, Ferrie and colleagues (2020) identified the desire of belongness with peers and a fear of social rejection as an overarching theme across studies. For instance, a child experiencing self-stigma may state, "*I am so embarrassing in front of other kids! My mental health challenges make me act so weird. They all must think I am so crazy* (stereotypes and prejudice). *I usually just hang out by myself at lunch and recess. I don't want to get made fun of* (discrimination)."

Self-stigma experienced by children with mental health challenges has been found to have negative emotional, psychosocial, behavioral, and health consequences. Higher levels of reported self-stigma by children with mental health challenges have been found to be related to diminished self-esteem, diminished feelings of self-efficacy, less willingness to engage in help-seeking, perceptions of loss-of control over symptoms, and increases in mental health symptoms (Ferrie, Miller, & Hunter, 2020; Keyes, Nolte, & Williams, 2018; Mitten et al., 2016; Moses, 2015; Rose et al., 2019). There are a variety of potential outcomes related to experiences of self-stigma, and the way the child copes has a notable influence on the impact of stigma (Ferrie, Miller, & Hunter, 2020; Moses, 2015). Children endorsing higher levels of self-stigma have been found to be more likely to endorse "disengagement coping" such as social avoidance and "disconfirming stereotypes" (i.e. attempts to compensate for or contradict negative stereotypes), are more likely to engage in label avoidance, and less likely to seek help (Ferrie, Miller, & Hunter, 2020; Keyes, Nolte, & Williams, 2018; Mitten et al., 2016; Moses, 2015; O'Connor et al., 2018).

As with adults with mental health challenges, there are a variety of ways that have been found to reduce the negative impacts of stigma. Knowledge regarding and acceptance of their mental health challenges, education regarding the stigma of mental health challenges, receiving support in response to disclosure, engaging in help-seeking, and social support have been found to reduce the negative impacts of self-stigma in children with mental health challenges (Ferrie, Miller, & Hunter, 2020; Keyes, Nolte, & Williams, 2018; Mitten et al., 2016; Moses, 2015; O'Connor et al., 2018). For instance, receiving education regarding mental health symptoms and receiving supportive responses to disclosure can help with "normalizing" the child's experiences, thus reducing feelings of "differentness" (i.e., combating negative stereotypes and prejudice).

Utilizing the social-cognitive model of stigma is useful for examining the stigma experiences of children with mental health challenges. Both public stigma and self-stigma can have negative impacts on targeted individuals. In summary, these stigma experiences can lead to losses of opportunities (e.g., less friendships) as well as negative emotional (e.g., low self-esteem), psychosocial (e.g., feelings different, disengagement coping), behavioral (e.g., less willingness to disclose or seek help), and health consequences (e.g., increase in mental health symptoms). Strategies exist that have potential to reduce negative consequences related to stigma that children with mental health challenges experience.

The stigma literature has historically focused on people with lived experience (i.e., adults and children with mental health challenges); however, experiences of stigma have been noted to cast a wide net and extend to others (Corrigan & Miller, 2004; Corrigan, Watson, & Miller, 2006; Moses, 2014; Perlick et al., 2011; Robinson & Brewster, 2016). Unlike adults, children are not independent. Minor children typically have some sort of parent/caregiver responsible for them. Having such a large role in their child's life, this begins to highlight the importance of extending the stigma literature in order to include experiences of parents/caregivers of children with mental health challenges.

2.3   Stigma Experienced by Parents/Caregivers

As stated earlier, experiences of public stigma have been found to extend from people with mental health challenges to their family members (Corrigan & Miller, 2004; Corrigan, Watson, & Miller, 2006; Goffman, 1963; Moses, 2014; Perlick et al., 2011; Phelan, Bromet, & Link, 1998; Robinson & Brewster, 2016; Shi et al., 2019; Tabatabaee, Yousefi Nooraie, Mohammad Aghaei, Rostam-Abadi, Sharifi, & Sharifi, 2023). In this particular context, the stigma associated with other family members has been labeled as family stigma, associative stigma, and courtesy stigma in the literature (Corrigan, Watson, & Miller, 2006; Eton, et al., 2016; Goffman, 1963; Mak & Cheung, 2008, 2012; Phelan, Bromet, & Link, 1998; Shi et al., 2019). This type of public stigma is defined as public stereotypes being extended to an individual due to their relationship to the person with mental health challenges (Eaton et al., 2016; Goffman, 1963; Moses, 2014).

Public stigma towards family members has been found to be related to feelings of shame, blame, and/or contamination (Corrigan & Miller, 2004; Corrigan, Watson, &

Miller, 2006). Research has noted that stigma experiences of family members varies by their role, finding differences between being the individual's parent, sibling, spouse/partner, or child (Corrigan & Miller, 2004; Corrigan, Watson, & Miller, 2006; Moses, 2014). For parents, others have been found to endorse blame (Corrigan & Miller, 2004; Corrigan, Watson, & Miller, 2006; McKeague et al., 2022; Moses, 2014; Weiner, 1995). In other words, people may think that the parent/caregiver is responsible for causing their child's mental health challenges. In action, parents/caregivers experiencing public stigma may be rejected by other parents/caregivers in the community and excluded from community events, teachers experiencing difficulties with their child at school who blame the parent may avoid offering support, or health care professionals may offer more limited treatment options due to blaming the parent/caregiver for the issues the child is experiencing. Public stigma can be viewed as a precursor to other forms of stigma experienced by parents, such as experiences of self-stigma and vicarious stigma (Corrigan & Wassel, 2008; Eaton et al., 2016; Moses, 2014). Abbreviated definitions and examples of the different forms of stigma discussed in this paper can be found in Table 1.

Table 1

Definitions and Examples of Stigma Experienced by Parents/Caregivers of Children with Mental Health Challenges

	Stigma Type		
	Public Stigma (Courtesy/Affiliate Stigma)	Self-Stigma	Vicarious Stigma
Definition	Endorsement of stereotypes and discrimination by public towards parents.	Parents internalize negative public stereotypes and discrimination.	Emotional response experienced by parents as a result of witnessing their child being stigmatized.
Stereotypes & Prejudice Example	"Those parents are responsible for their child's mental health challenges …they should feel ashamed of themselves!"	"I'm such a bad parent…I can't even control my own child."	"I am so upset watching my child get teased and excluded by others at soccer practice because of their mental health challenges."
Discrimination Example	Community members exclude family from the annual BBQ.	Parent does not attend family gatherings.	Parent removes their child from the practice and decides to quit the soccer team.

2.3.1   Self-Stigma Experienced by Parents/Caregivers. Just as adults and children

with mental health challenges internalize stigma and experience feelings of shame,

parents/caregivers of children with mental health challenges have a similar experience.

Parents/caregivers of children with mental health challenges experience self-stigma when

they become aware of stereotypes towards themselves, and then internalize these views

as their own (Perlick et al., 2011). For instance, parents/caregivers may internalize and

agree with public beliefs of blame, and in turn, blame themselves for their children's

mental health challenges. For example, a parent/caregiver experiencing self-stigma may say, *"I am so ashamed, it is all my fault that my child struggles with mental health challenges."* These feelings of self-blame have been related to diminished psychological wellbeing in parents/caregivers of children with mental health challenges (Moses, 2010). A study examining the pathway of self-stigma experienced by parents of children with mental health challenges by Eaton and colleagues (2020) found significant direct pathways from stigma awareness, to self-doubt, to self-stigma, to affective distress.

To reiterate, research examining people with mental health challenges has demonstrated a link between experiences of self-stigma and diminished feelings of self-esteem and self-efficacy (Corrigan, Watson, & Barr, 2006; Drapalski et al., 2013; Watson et al., 2007). Studies examining parents/caregivers of children with mental health challenges have been consistent with the literature regarding individuals with lived experience – where self-stigma has been found to negatively impact feelings of self-esteem and self-efficacy (Corrigan, Watson, & Miller, 2006; Eaton at al., 2016; Hasson-Ohayon et al., 2019). Self-efficacy for parents/caregivers in this context is believing that they are capable of successfully performing their roles as a parent/caregiver (Coleman & Karraker, 2003; Li et al., 2019; Murdock, 2013). Parents/caregivers experiences of self-stigma may lead to a diminished sense of being a "good parent," which can be extremely distressing (Chan & Lam, 2017; Corrigan et al., 2016; Corrigan, Watson, & Miller, 2006; Eaton at al., 2016; Moses, 2014). Some parents/caregivers have also been found to endorse common public beliefs of incompetence, and in turn, respond by concealing their child's mental health challenges in attempts to protect themselves from discomfort and/or rejection (Chan & Lam, 2018; Struening et al., 2001; Zisman-Ilani et al., 2013).

As noted earlier, potential consequences of disclosing mental health challenges may include blame, disapproval, and avoidance by others (Corrigan & Matthews, 2003). Thus, deciding whether to disclose mental health challenges or conceal them can be a difficult decision to make for parents/caregivers of children with mental health challenges (Homes & River, 1998; Corrigan & Matthews, 2003). Parents/caregivers of children with mental health challenges who are experiencing high levels of self-stigma may be more likely to opt for concealment or secrecy coping over disclosure (Corrigan & Matthews, 2003; Link et al., 1997; Luoma et al., 2007). The potential negative consequences are important for parents/caregivers to consider; however, disclosure of mental health challenges has the capability of reducing negative impacts of perceived stigma such as reducing stigma-related distress as well as facilitate support for the parent and/or their child with mental health challenges (Corrigan et al., 2010; Corrigan et al., 2012). For instance, a parent/caregiver who is willing to disclose may have more opportunities to meet other parents/caregivers who have children with similar mental health challenges. Having open conversations about their lived experience with others, this parent/caregiver may be invited to attend a support group with other parents/caregivers and/or is able to find appropriate referrals for services. Hearing and learning from other parents'/caregivers' experiences parenting a child with mental health challenges has the potential to reduce the self-stigmatizing attitudes of blame and incompetence the parent/caregiver may be endorsing as well.

2.3.2 Vicarious Stigma Experienced by Parents/Caregivers. There are additional components to stigma uniquely related to the experiences of family members related to an individual with mental health challenges. Vicarious stigma can be defined as the emotional response experienced by an individual as a result of witnessing the stigmatization of another relative/loved one (Corrigan & Miller, 2004; Serchuk, Corrigan, Reed, & Ohan, 2021). In other words, a parent/caregiver may experience a negative emotional response from witnessing the stigmatization of their child with mental health challenges. Parents have been found to suffer when they observe their child with mental health challenges experiencing stigma (Corrigan & Miller, 2004; Robinson & Brrewster, 2016; Struening et al., 2001; Wahl & Harman, 1989). Previous research has found vicarious stigma experienced by parents/caregivers to have a relation with negative emotional outcomes (Chan & Leung, 2021; Eaton et al., 2016; Robinson & Brewster, 2016; Serchuk et al., 2021).

Vicarious stigma is a relatively new area of study, and little is empirically known regarding its effects. A related concept, vicarious experience, is when an individual has an empathic response to observing another's affect and/or behavior (Keysers & Gazzola, 2009). Research has indicated that for particular sensations, emotions, and actions, one's vicarious experience of a situation has similar neurological processes as if it were that individual's primary experience (Keysers & Gazzola, 2009; Jackson, Meltzoff, & Decety, 2005; Morrison et al., 2004). As mentioned earlier, a common form of discrimination experienced by children with mental health challenges can come in the form of bullying by their peers (Moses, 2010). A review examining the experiences of parents of children who have been bullied found common themes of negative emotional responses across studies, including feelings of anger, guilt, frustration, stress, and worry (Harcourt, Jasperse, & Green, 2014). More research is needed to more fully understand the relatively novel concept of vicarious stigma.

To this date, there are only two psychometrically tested measures that specifically include vicarious stigma as a construct. The Lesbian, Gay, Bisexual Affiliate Stigma Measure (LGM-ASM) was developed by Robinson and Brewster (2016) to examine the stigma experienced by heterosexual family and close friends of LGB individuals. This measure demonstrated good internal consistencies and test-retest reliabilities, and the factor structure was determined by exploratory factor analysis (EFA) and confirmatory factor analysis (CFA). The final LGB-ASM included 17-items across three factors – public discrimination/rejection affiliate stigma, vicarious affiliate stigma, public shame affiliate stigma (Robinson & Brewster, 2016). To measure vicarious stigma in the current investigation, a fairly new measure called the Vicarious Stigma Scale was used. This scale was created to measure vicarious stigma specifically experienced by parents/caregivers of a child with mental health challenges. This measure utilized community-based participatory research (e.g., qualitative interviews with parents/caregivers of children with mental health challenges were used to create/inform the measure), and based on the literature and qualitative investigation, this measure examines vicarious stigma related to two emotional responses - sadness and anger. Previous research on The Vicarious Stigma Scale demonstrated good internal consistency and an EFA conducted found support for the two-factor structure of sadness of anger (more information can be found in subsection 3.5 Measures; Serchuk, Corrigan, Reed, and Ohan, 2021). The proposed study will add to the existing literature by further exploring vicarious stigma experienced by parents/caregivers of minor children by utilizing a measure created for this specific population. The proposed study will further examine the psychometric properties of this vicarious stigma measure, which may facilitate examining vicarious stigma experienced by this population in future studies.

2.4   Impact of Stigma on Parents/Caregivers

Aspects of public stigma, self-stigma, and vicarious stigma have been found to have various impacts on parents/caregivers of children with mental health challenges. This section will discuss literature examining the experiences of stigma by parents/caregivers of children with mental health challenges and how it relates to symptoms of depression and help-seeking (Corrigan, Druss, & Perlick, 2014; Moses, 2014; Muralidharan et al., 2016; Vogel, Wade, & Hackler, 2007). A summary of the impacts of stigma on outcome variables are depicted below. When directed at the parent/caregiver or their child with mental health challenges, public stigma can lead to a loss of opportunities (e.g., less supports). As seen in Figure 3, when public stigma directed at the parent/caregiver is agreed with and internalized (i.e., experience self-stigma), they may endorse common feelings of shame and blame, which may lead to increased symptoms of depression and negative attitudes towards help-seeking.

Figure 3

Summary of The Impacts of Public Stigma and Self-Stigma on Depression and Help-Seeking

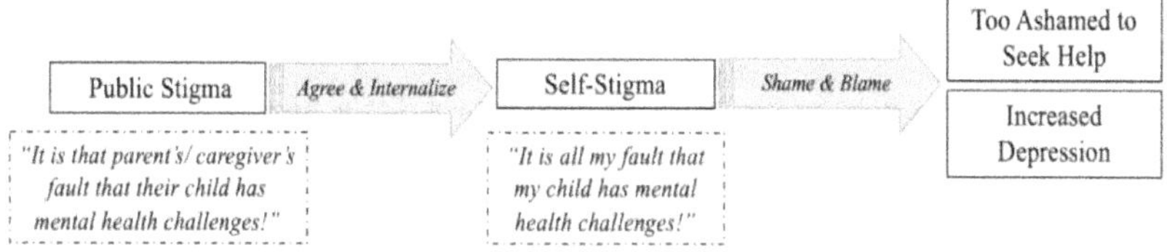

As seen in Figure 4, when a parent/caregiver witnesses public stigma directed at the child with mental health challenges, the parent/caregiver may have feelings of sadness and/or anger from experiencing vicarious stigma, which may lead to increased symptoms of depression and more willingness to seek-help.

Figure 4

Summary of The Impacts of Public Stigma and Vicarious Stigma on Depression and Help-Seeking

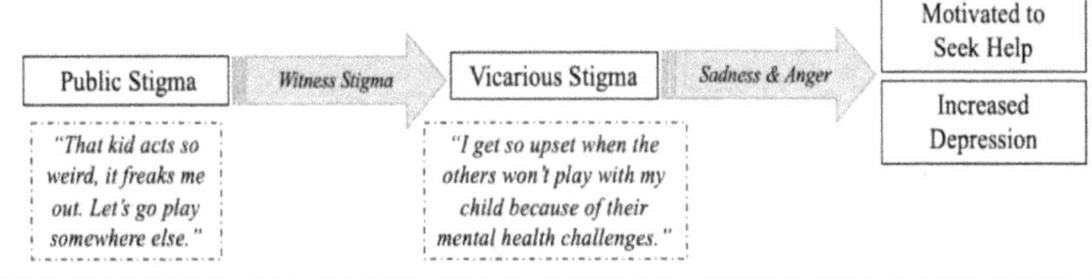

2.4.1 Stigma and Depression. The stigma experienced by a parent/caregiver of a child with mental health challenges has been linked to symptoms of depression such as sadness, rumination, and feelings of guilt (Cantwell, Muldoon, & Gallagher, 2015; Chan, Fung, & Leunh, 2022; Eaton et al., 2016; Eaton et al., 2020; Mercando et al., 2020; Mickalson, 2001; Moses, 2010, 2014; Öz et al., 2020; Shi et al., 2019; Singh, 2004; Stengler-Wenzke, Trosbach, Dietrich, & Angermeyer, 2004). Emotional wellbeing, which includes levels of depression, of a parent/caregiver is known to have a noteworthy influence on their child's emotional and behavioral development (Bayer et al., 2019; Blesky, 1984; Brennan et al., 2000; Dreyer et al., 2018; Edwards, Rapee, & Kennedy, 2010; Eton et al., 2016; Gottman, Katz, & Hooven, 1996; Moses, 2014). This further highlights the importance of studying the emotional impact of stigma experienced by parents/caregivers for the sake of the parents/caregivers as well as their children.

There has recently been an influx in literature demonstrating significant pathways between depression and types of stigma experienced by parents/caregivers of children with mental health challenges. In a study examining 424 parents of children with mental health challenges, significant direct pathways were found from awareness of public stigma, to self-doubt, to self-stigma, to affective distress which included symptoms of depression (Eaton et al., 2020). These findings add to the literature, such that examining the stigma experiences and related outcomes for parents/caregivers of minor children with mental health challenges. Measurement of "affective distress" in this study examined parent symptoms of depression and anxiety. The proposed study hopes to add to the research examining parent/caregiver symptoms related specifically to depression. The "stigma awareness" and "self-doubt" variables in this study were measured utilizing items created for the study, adapted from qualitative research. In other words, a significant weakness identified in this study includes utilizing unvalidated "measures" to assess 2 key variables explored. The proposed study adds to the literature, specifically examining parental self-stigma, by incorporating measures of public stigma awareness that have been used previously and have been found to have good psychometric properties. In line with the proposed study, Eaton and colleagues (2020) had utilized the same, fairly new, measure of parent self-stigma. The proposed study will add to the growing knowledge of the psychometric properties of this measure, which will hopefully facilitate examining parental self-stigma in future studies.

In a study of 400 caregivers for children with a diagnosis with ADHD, Chen and colleagues (2021) found a significant positive relation between affiliate stigma and levels of depression, which were moderated by family support (negative relation), self-esteem (negative relation), and child symptomatology (positive relation). A significant strength of this study includes recruiting parents of children who were receiving services at outpatient clinics, and ADHD (e.g., child diagnosis) was determined via diagnostic clinical interview and observations. Chen and colleagues (2021) also utilized the same measure of parental/caregiver depression proposed for this study, which can allow for future comparison. This study, however, was constrained to parents of children with a specific diagnosis and did not include a measure of parental self-stigma. The proposed study hopes to expand the generalizability of results by including parents/caregivers of children who can present with a variety of different mental health challenges, and the study will add to the literature by incorporating a measure of parental self-stigma.

Additionally, the proposed study further adds to the literature regarding the new concept of vicarious stigma, which was not examined in either of the above studies mentioned (Chen et al., 2021; Eaton et al., 2020). In a study of 441 parents of children with autism spectrum disorder, Chan and Leung (2021) examined a mediation model connecting higher child symptomatology to higher levels of depression symptoms reported by parents via two significant pathways: (1) perceptions of public stigma towards their child and vicarious stigma, and (2) perceptions of public stigma towards parents of children with autism spectrum disorder and self-stigma. In other words, significant positive pathways were found from child symptoms, to experiences of public stigma towards the child, to vicarious stigma, to depression symptoms; and significant positive pathway from child symptoms, to experiences of public stigma towards parents of children with autism spectrum disorder, to self-stigma, to depression symptoms. A significant strength of this study is confirming child diagnosis by recruiting from specialized schools and service centers for autism, and assessing children by a licensed clinician. However, most of the children in this sample were diagnosed with a comorbid intellectual disability; which the article noted could limit generalizability. The proposed study hopes to add to the limited literature examining the differential effects of public stigma directed towards the child versus their parent/caregiver, and how that related to parent/caregiver experiences of self-stigma and vicarious stigma. Further, Chan and Leung (2021) adapted a fairly new measure of vicarious stigma originally developed for examining affiliate stigma experienced by family and close friends of adults identifying as lesbian, gay, or bisexual (Robinson & Brewster, 2016). The proposed study will add to the existing literature by further exploring vicarious stigma experienced by parents/caregivers of minor children by utilizing a measure created for this specific population and further examining the psychometric properties of this vicarious stigma measure, which may facilitate examining vicarious stigma experienced by this population in future studies. Further, each of the studies mentioned above were constrained to specific countries/cities (e.g., Australia and New Zealand, Hong Kong, Taiwan). The proposed study will be recruiting participants via an online crowdsourcing website – where participants can be potentially located in a variety of countries from around the world. Thus, results from the proposed study may be more generalizable due to a potentially broad range of backgrounds.

Based on the information presented, an example of a parent/caregiver experiencing self-stigma may report, *"It's my fault my child still cannot take the bus to school without having a panic attack. I feel so sad and guilty thinking about how I have to drive my child to school every day because of my bad parenting!"* Experiencing the effects of vicarious stigma, the parent/caregiver mentioned above may say, *"The other day my child was not allowed to attend an assembly at school because their teacher wanted to avoid having to deal with a potential panic attack. My child needs a little more support and could have attended the assembly without disturbing other students if they were given their accommodations. How often has my child been getting excluded because of their anxiety? ...I can't stop thinking about it, I've been up crying at night."* An aim of this study will be to examine the relation between levels of public stigma, self-stigma, and vicarious stigma with levels of depression symptoms experienced by parents/caregivers of children with mental health challenges.

2.4.2   Stigma and Help-Seeking. Experiences of stigma may also undermine help-seeking attitudes and behavior of parents/caregivers of children with mental health challenges. Research has indicated that more than half of children with mental health challenges in the United States do not receive treatment for their mental health challenges and related problems (Merikangas et al., 2010; Olfson et al., 2014; Whitney & Paterson, 2019). Parents/caregivers are crucial in their child's ability to access mental health services, and they often act as gatekeepers (Reardon et al., 2018; Villatoro et al., 2018). Literature reviews have identified common barriers to seeking help endorsed by parents/caregivers of children with mental health challenges including structural issues (e.g., treatment affordability, issues with transportation), knowledge and recognition of mental health challenges, attitudes towards mental health treatment, understanding of the help-seeking process, and family/social factors (Planey et al., 2019; Radez et al., 2021; Reardon et al., 2017; Reardon et al., 2018).

As mentioned earlier, pubic stigma may be endorsed by family, friends, teachers, doctors, and other individuals. When a parent/caregiver typically seeks advice or help with something related to their child, there are usually a variety of helpful options available.

However, when a parent/caregiver of a child with mental health challenges seeks help, it can be more difficult to find helpful, non-judgmental assistance and support. Family members often report strained and distant relationships with friends and/or extended family because of a relative with mental health challenges and the stigma involved (Corrigan & Miller, 2004; Östman & Kjellin, 2002; Shibre et al., 2001; Struening et al., 2001; Tabatabaee et al., 2023; Wahl & Harman, 1989). Family members may also consider their relationship to a person with mental health challenges as a source of shame to the family that should be hidden, which is a form of public stigma (Angermeyer, Schulze, & Dietrich, 2003; Ohaeri & Fido, 2001; Phelan, Bromet, & Link, 1998; Phillips, et al., 2002; Shibre et al., 2001; Thompson & Doll, 1982; Wahl & Harman, 1989). Further, research on adults with mental health challenges has found that their attitudes regarding help-seeking is related to the opinions, past experiences, and recommendations of their friends and family (Angermeyer, Matschinger, & Riedel-Heller, 2001; Planey et al., 2019; Vogel, Wade, Wester, Larson, & Hackler, 2007). In a study of 3,149 adults, Villatoro and Aneshensel (2014) found that individuals reported more willingness to seek mental health services for their child when they perceived lower levels of stigmatizing attitudes from their family.

Research has found that stigma related to mental health challenges can act as a significant barrier to help-seeking (Clement et al., 2015; Corrigan, 2004; Corrigan, Druss, & Perlick, 2014; Villatoro et al., 2018). Individuals with mental health challenges who report experiencing higher levels of self-stigma have been found to endorse negative attitudes towards help-seeking (Conceição, Rothes, & Gusmão, 2021; Dempster et al., 2015; Dempster et al., 2013; Conner et al., 2010; Jung, von Sternberg, & Davis, 2017; Reardon et al., 2017; Vogel, Wade, & Hackler, 2007) as well as have lower levels of treatment adherence (Carrara & Ventura, 2018; Tong et al., 2020). Parents/caregivers of children with mental health challenges experiencing self-stigma may endorse common public beliefs of blame and/or incompetence, and in turn, respond by avoiding or delaying engagement in help-seeking behaviors (Corrigan, 2004; Dempster et al., 2015; Dempster et al., 2013; Struening et al., 2001; Tucker et al., 2013; Zisman-Ilani et al., 2013).

Overall, public stigma limits options for help-seeking, and has the potential to perpetuate self-stigma experienced by parents/caregivers. In a study of adults with mental health challenges, Vogel, Wade, and Hackler (2007) found that perceptions of public stigma had a positive relation with self-stigma, and levels of self-stigma were negatively related to attitudes towards help-seeking. Self-stigma was found to be a significant mediator of the relationship between public stigma and help-seeking attitudes in the study (Vogel, Wade, & Hackler, 2007). In other words, individuals who endorsed experiencing higher levels of public stigma and self-stigma felt more negatively towards help-seeking. A parent seeking help for their child may experience self-stigma, blaming themselves and/or their parenting for their child's mental health challenges and related difficulties (Corrigan et al., 2016; Corrigan, Watson, & Miller, 2006; Eaton et al., 2016; Moses, 2014). The proposed study aims to replicate these findings in a population of parents/caregivers of children with mental health challenges, and examining the negative relation public and self-stigma has with attitudes towards help-seeking for themselves as well as for their child.

To this date, the existing literature examining experiences of vicarious stigma have not included help-seeking as a variable of interest. The proposed study hopes to add to the existing literature on parent/caregiver sigma experiences broadly, and more specifically exploring the novel concept of vicarious stigma. The negative role of public stigma and self-stigma on help-seeking in a population of adults with mental health challenges has been well documented, and there has been research generally exploring these variables in parents/caregivers of children with mental health challenges. The proposed study hopes to replicate these findings and take a deeper dive into help-seeking by specifying attitudes towards help-seeking for themselves and also for their child in a population of parents/caregivers of children with mental health challenges. Utilizing a sample of participants that demonstrates this relationship between public stigma, self-stigma, and help-seeking consistent with previous research provides a good opportunity for examining the fairly new construct of vicarious stigma. As mentioned previously, vicarious stigma has been conceptualized in this context as the empathetic response of sadness and/or anger experienced by a parent/caregiver when witnessing the stigmatization of their child with mental health challenges (Corrigan & Miller, 2004; Keysers & Gazzola, 2009; Serchuk et al., 2021). Also, research has noted different responses to perceptions of stigma – unaffected, internalized and suffer negative consequences, and "righteous indignation" and feelings of personal empowerment (Corrigan & Rao, 2012). While self-stigma occurs when individuals become aware of, agree with, and internalize public stereotypes (Corrigan & Watson, 2002), it may be possible that parents/caregivers of children with mental health challenges respond to vicarious stigma in line with feelings of "righteous indignation," recognizing the injustice of stigma experienced by their child. Having an emotional reaction to witnessing their child experiencing stigma (i.e., vicarious stigma), parents/caregivers may feel energized to take action; in contrast to isolation and avoidance related with experiencing self-stigma. Thus, the current proposal hypothesizes that experiencing higher levels of vicarious stigma will have a direct relation with more favorable attitudes towards help-seeking for their child.

Based on the information presented, an example of a parent/caregiver experiencing high levels of self-stigma may report, "*I messed up my kid so bad, I am too ashamed to ask for help.*" Experiencing high levels of vicarious stigma, a parent/caregiver may report, "*I get so upset watching my child get in trouble at school because of their mental health challenges. I am going to call the school tomorrow to see if my child can receive additional support!*" This study will also aim to examine the relation between levels of public stigma, self-stigma, and vicarious stigma with help-seeking by parents/caregivers of children with mental health challenges.

2.5   Summary of Hypotheses

As shown in the path model (Figure 1), this study proposed to examine the role of public, self- and vicarious stigma in relation to symptoms of depression and help-seeking. It was predicted that public stigmas will be related with all variables of interest, and will act as a precursor to self- and vicarious stigma in the model. Both self-stigma and vicarious stigma experienced by parents were predicted to have independent relations with the outcome variables.

An additional pursuit of this investigation will be to further examine the psychometric properties and factor structure of The Vicarious Stigma Scale, which was utilized to measure vicarious stigma in this study. As mentioned above, there are limited measures created specifically to examine stigma in a population of parents/caregivers of children with mental health challenges and the concept of vicarious stigma is a relatively new area of study. The Vicarious Stigma Scale was developed specifically for parents/caregivers of children with mental health challenges utilizing community-based participatory research and has gone through limited psychometric testing (more information can be found in subsection 3.5 Measures). Thus, this investigation will add to the research examining this novel scale of vicarious stigma.

H1: Public stigma towards parents/caregivers of children with mental health challenges will be positively related with self-stigma and depression

H2: Public stigma towards people with mental health challenges will be positively related with vicarious stigma and depression.

H3: Public stigma towards parents/caregivers of children with mental health challenges will be negatively related to attitudes towards help-seeking for themselves and attitudes towards help-seeking for their child with mental health challenges

H4: Self-stigma will be positively related to vicarious stigma and depression

H5: Self-stigma will be negatively related to attitudes towards help-seeking for themselves and attitudes towards help-seeking for their child with mental health challenges

H6: Vicarious stigma will be positively related to depression and attitudes towards help-seeking for their child with mental health challenges

H7: The relationship between public stigma towards parents/caregivers, help-seeking for their child and for themselves, and depression will be mediated by self-stigma

H8: The relationship between public stigma towards people with mental health challenges, help-seeking for their child, and depression will be mediated by vicarious stigma

Figure 1

Hypothesized Model (repeated from Chapter 1)

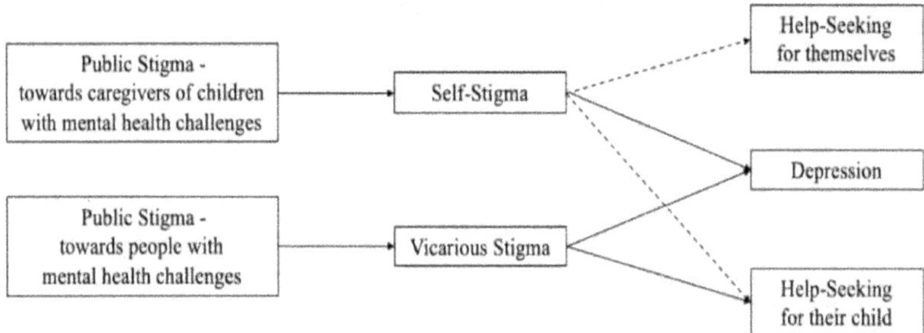

Note. Dashed line indicates negative relationship.

CHAPTER 3

METHOD

3.1   Overview

The current investigation included two components – first, a qualitative

investigation, and then second, a quantitative investigation. The qualitative investigation

involved interviewing a small number of stakeholders in order to inform recruitment

materials and survey questions for the quantitative investigation. Utilizing this form of

community-based participatory research enhances the content validity of questions

informed by the qualitative interviews. The quantitative component of this project will

then investigate the aims and hypotheses summarized above.

3.2   Participants

Both components of the investigation (qualitative and quantitative) utilized the

same criteria for participants. For inclusion in the study, participants must be at least 18

years of age and indicate that they are a parent/caregiver of a minor child (age 3-18) with

diagnosed mental health challenges. For the purposes of this study, *mental health*

challenges will refer to internalizing problems (e.g., anxiety disorders, depressive

disorders), externalizing problems (e.g., disruptive behavior problems, oppositional

defiant disorder), and/or neurodevelopmental disorders (e.g., attention-

deficit/hyperactivity disorder, autism spectrum disorder). Children as young as 3-years-

old may be included because literature indicates that symptoms of many of the disorders

included can first appear at this age or earlier (Hopkins, Lavigne, Gouze, LeBailly, &

Bryant, 2013; Lavigne, LeBailly, Hopkins, Gouze & Binns, 2009). For the purposes of this study, the term "parent/caregiver" will refer to the custodial parent or adult legally responsible for a child, and this can include biological parent and adoptive parents.

Study exclusion criteria included parent/caregivers who identify their child as having been diagnosed with an intellectual disability. This exclusion criterion was based on previous research utilizing community-based participatory research interviews, which revealed that parents of children with this type of disability have been found to endorse different experiences of stigma (e.g., more pity) compared to parents of children with other mental health challenges (e.g., parent-blame) (Ditchman et al., 2013; Eaton, Ohan, Stritzke, & Corrigan, 2019; Mak & Cheung, 2008). There are notable rates of comorbidity between autism spectrum disorder and intellectual disability diagnoses. Parents of children with autism spectrum disorder, who also deny the presence of a comorbid diagnosis of intellectual disability, were included since they were found to have similar, parent-blaming experiences of stigma.

3.3   Procedures

Participants were recruited via Prolific (www.prolific.co), an online crowdsourcing platform that can be utilized for recruiting participants for research studies. Studies have shown that Prolific may be a better option compared to other popular online crowdsourcing recruitment platforms such as MTurk (Palan & Schitter, 2018; Peer et al., 2017; Peer et al., 2021). Some advantages to utilizing Prolific for recruitment include high data quality and having access to a diverse pool of naïve participants (i.e., participants who are less familiar with common experimental research tasks) (Palan & Schitter, 2018; Peer et al., 2017; Peer et al., 2021).

Users on Prolific provide a variety of demographic data, which can be utilized as a pre-screening filter. For example, Prolific stated that there are 31,219 participants who have been active within the last 90-days who fit the following criteria: fluent in English and reported that they have a child. The demographic prescreening tool was helpful in restraining the recruitment audience, however, could not ensure that the parent's/caregiver's child is (1) aged 3-18 and (2) has mental health challenges.

Of note, Prolific has regulations regarding participant compensation – one of these being that all participants who respond to a survey must be compensated, regardless of meeting study exclusionary criteria (i.e., a participant who gets screened-out of a survey after a few questions due to ineligibility must be compensated the same amount as an eligible participant who completes the full study). In order to recruit a more specific sample while following the platform regulations, the Prolific Help Centre recommended creating a 2-part study – consisting of (part 1) a short screener survey to capture relevant demographic components of interested participants, and then (part 2) inviting only the eligible participants to the main survey utilizing the "custom allowlist" tool. Thus, a screener survey was necessary and was created to identify eligible participants for each component of the study.

Thus, screening the participants was completed via Prolific's embedded "demographic prescreening" tool, and a separate set of screener questions on Qualtrics were used to assess eligibility (Appendix A). Then, the qualitative interview/quantitative survey became available if inclusion criteria were met (Figure5).

Figure 5

Timeline of Data Collection

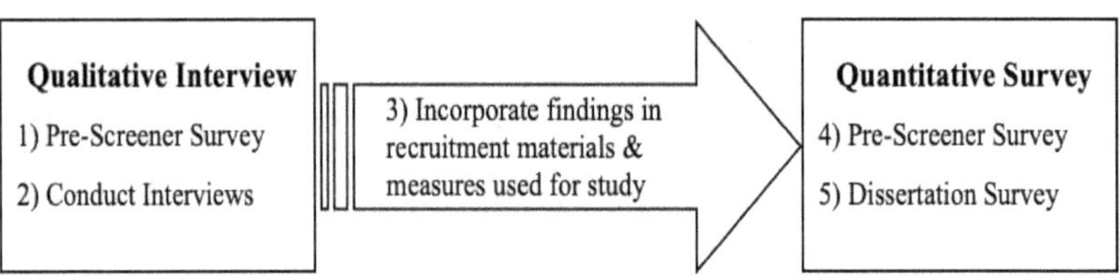

In order to further ensure quality data, an attention check question was presented during the quantitative survey. Prolific requires payment per minute, participant compensation will be calculated based on the U.S. federal minimum wage of $7.25. Parents/caregivers were compensated $0.42 for completing the qualitative interview screener survey, and those who completed the approximately 30-minute qualitative interview were compensated with $4.75 and a $15 Amazon gift card. Parents/caregivers who completed the quantitative pre-screening survey were compensated $0.32, and those who were eligible and completed the larger quantitative survey were compensated $3.03. Participants spent an average of 13.18 minutes (*standard deviation* = 8.09 minutes) completing the survey questions on the larger dissertation survey. The total cost of this investigation, including participant compensation and Prolific fees, was $1392.50 USD.

3.4   Qualitative Investigation

The qualitative interviews were conducted with N=5 stakeholders – which included service providers (n=2) and parents/caregivers of children with mental health challenges (as defined above) (n=3) in order to clarify language used in this study. The qualitative investigation was an important and useful component to this investigation;

however, it was not a main focus of the overall project. Thus, a small sample was collected for the qualitative investigation.

Specific words of concern included "diagnosis," "primary caregiver," and "mental health challenges." The qualitative interviews with parents/caregivers were conducted via telephone utilizing a pre-determined set of open-ended questions, which can be found in Appendix A. Participants were provided a link to a document in order to follow along with verbally presented questions. The qualitative interview began with questions intended to be about the child (questions 1-5), followed by questions intended to be about the parent/caregiver (6-7), and then questions from a measure of public stigma (8-9). Parents/caregivers were asked if they understood various words/phrases used in questions, and if they had suggestions or preferences for other words. Participants verbally responded to the interviewer's queries regarding the presented questions. Interviewer took notes regarding participant responses. The interviews with service providers were conducted verbally in person. Once the qualitative data was collected, it was examined for common themes. Results from the interviews informed the language used in recruiting materials and survey questions for the quantitative investigation.

3.4.1 Description of Qualitative Sample. The 3 Prolific participants were female, age range was 24-44 years, were all fluent English speakers. Participants identified as a primary caregiver of 1-3 minor children with mental health challenges. Reported child diagnoses included anxiety, depression, and ADHD. 1 parent reported that they have a mental health diagnosis, 1 participant denied, and 1 participant did not want to answer. Each participant was located in a different geographical region of the United States.

Additionally, 2 services providers located in the United States participated in interviews. The service providers included a licensed pediatric clinical psychologist (PhD) at a large academic medical center and a Master's level school psychologist at an elementary school setting. Both service providers are also currently active researchers in the field of clinical psychology.

3.4.1   Summary of Qualitative Findings. Overall, the interviewer observed significant similarity in responses across participants. A more detailed summary of responses to each question presented during the interviews can be found in Appendix B. All participants understood and agreed with the phrases "primary caregiver" and "diagnosis." Participants confirmed that diagnoses and treatments presented in demographic questions were representative and inclusive. Suggestions included shortening demographic questions and adding examples of common mental health challenges at the beginning of measures for clarification.

Consulting with stakeholders helped the interviewer create a short list of phrases that could be used to potentially replace "mental health challenges." The 3 parent-participants reported a preference for the phrase "social, emotional, and/or behavioral difficulties." Thus, all recruitment materials and survey questions utilized the phrase.

Regarding a question from the measure of public stigma containing the phrase "mental hospital." All parents endorsed understanding the phrase "mental hospital," however, they each mentioned that this term is not used frequently and may not be the most representative phrase. Participant suggestions included "mental health facility," "mental health treatment program," "psychiatric ward," and "in-patient facility." Although parents indicated potentially more representative phrases, the interviewer noted that each parent seemed to feel negatively about the phrase. Of note, this measure of public stigma is already undergoing other adaptations to wording for this project. Since "mental hospital" was understood by all parents, the phrase "mental hospital" was retained in order to maintain the integrity of the measure.

Results from the qualitative interviews with people with lived experience and service providers were used to inform recruitment materials and questionnaires for the larger dissertation project. Overall, minor changes to wording/phrases were indicated.

3.5   Measures

The present study included measures of demographic factors, public stigma, self-stigma, vicarious stigma, help-seeking, and depression. The measures used are provided in Appendix A, which incorporate adaptations to wording based on the qualitative interviews. A summary of measurement details and Cronbach's alphas computed from the sample of this study can be found in Table 2.

Demographic factors measured for this study included items about the parent/caregiver participant and their child with mental health challenges. This included a short screener questionnaire that asked for the parent and child's age and other relevant questions for determining inclusion in the study. Data from the screener and the larger demographics measure were used as a quality control check (e.g., compare consistency of demographic data across surveys). Items about the parent included age, gender, ethnicity, race, marital status, employment status, approximate family income, highest level of education achieved, history of mental health challenges and treatment, number of children they have that have been diagnosed with mental health challenges, and the relationship to their child. Items about their child included age, gender, race, ethnicity, diagnoses, primary diagnosis, approximate year of diagnosis, professional who provided the diagnosis, and current treatments/supports the child is currently receiving.

Public stigma was measured using adapted versions of the Devaluation of Consumers Who Have Serious Mental Illness and Devaluation of Families of Consumers Who Have Serious Mental Illness scales (Struening, Perlick, Link, Hellman, Herman, & Sirey, 2001). Together, these scales are 15 items scored on a 4-point Likert scale (1=strongly disagree to 4=strongly agree). The Devaluation of Customers scale is 8 items examining public stigma endorsed towards people with mental illness, which has demonstrated good internal consistency (α = .82) (Struening et al., 2001). The Devaluation of Families scale has 7 items examining public/curtesy stigma towards the families of people with mental illness, which has demonstrated adequate internal consistency (α = .71-.77) (Struening et al., 2001). These scales have previously been adapted specifically for studies examining families of people with autism spectrum disorder (ASD), and have reported good internal consistencies for both the adapted Devaluation of Customers scale (α = .83) the adapted Devaluation of Families (α = .86-.89) scales (Chan et al., 2017; Mak & Kwok, 2010). For example, original item *"Most people look down on families that have a member who is mentally ill living with them"* was changed to *"Most people look down on families who have a member who has an ASD"* in the study by Chan et al (2017). Adaptations to items for this study was based on adaptations previously made in the literature, and specific wording choices made were based on the results of the qualitative interviews. Thus, the original item from the measure will be adapted to, *"Most people look down on parents who have a child with social, emotional, and/or behavioral difficulties,"* for the purposes of this study.

Self-stigma was measured using the Parents' Self-Stigma Scale (PSSS; Eaton et al., 2019), which assesses the degree to which parents of children with mental health challenges experience self-stigma. This 11-item, self-report measure asks participants to rate each item on a 5-point scale (1=never to 5=almost all the time) (e.g., *"The way I have raised my child has contributed to his/her problem"*). Higher scores represent higher levels of self-stigma. The PSSS has demonstrated good internal consistency (α = .84) and evidence for convergent validity with other measures of related constructs (r = .34-.57) (Eaton et al., 2019).

Vicarious stigma was measured using The Vicarious Stigma Scale, created for a larger study based on experience and qualitative investigations with parents of children with mental health challenges. Development of this scale utilized community-based participatory research, enhancing the content validity of this measure. Serchuk, Corrigan, Reed, and Ohan (2021) utilized the original 14-item Vicarious Stigma Scale, and conducted an exploratory factor analysis (EFA) with a Varimax rotation in a population of parents of children with mental health challenges and/or neurodevelopmental disorders. The Kaiser-Meyer-Olkin (KMO) measure was .64 and Bartlett's test of sphericity was found to be statistically significant (p = .000), supporting the validity of the EFA. The EFA indicated a 2-factor solution for the scale, with 12 items total. The Vicarious Stigma Scale asks participants to rate agreement on a 10-point scale (1 = not at all to 10 = extremely so) across 2 dimensions: sadness (6 items) and anger (6 items). There is an "N/A" option for each item, used if the participant has not experienced the situation. Scores will be computed by calculating the items for the sadness and anger sub-scales, as well as an overall vicarious stigma score. Higher scores indicate experiencing higher levels of vicarious stigma. Since this measure was developed for a larger study still in progress, psychometric properties are limited. Internal consistency of the 12-item scale has been satisfactory for each scale (sadness α = .78; anger α = .79) (Serchuk et al., 2021).

Depression was measured using The Center for Epidemiological Studies Short Depression Scale (CESD-R-10; Anderson et al., 1994). The CESD-R-10 assess parents' feelings of being down or depressed over the last week. This 10-item, self-report measure asks participants to first "check" items that apply (e.g., "*I felt depressed*") and then indicate frequency using a rating scale (rarely or none of the times (less than 1 day) to all of the time (5-7 days)). Higher scores represent greater levels of depression symptoms. Previous research on the CES-D-10 has demonstrated good internal consistency (α = .81-.89), good construct validity correlations with similar constructs (r = .57-.86), and good test-retest reliability (r = .21-.84) (Anderson et al., 1994; Anderson et al., 2013; Björgvinsson et al., 2013; Miller, Anton, & Townson, 2008).

Help-seeking behaviors was measured using The General Help-Seeking Questionnaire (GHSQ; Wilson et al., 2005). The GHSQ was created as a flexible measure of help-seeking attitudes from professional and non-professional sources adapted for parents of children with mental health challenges for the purposes of this study (e.g., instructions will be presented twice with the original prompt as well as an adapted prompt - Original: "*If you were having a problem, how likely is it that you seek help or support from the following people/sources?*" and Adapted: "*If your child were having a problem, how likely is it that you seek help or support from the following people/sources?"*). Items assess help-seeking attitudes from 10 different sources (e.g., partner, friend, doctor, teacher). The first 10 items ask participants how likely they would be to ask for help or support from each source on a 7-point Likert scale (1 = extremely unlikely to 7 = extremely likely; "N/A" for "not applicable" will appear for parents' who do not have that source available). The last item states, "I would not seek help," which was reversed scored. The 11 items will be repeated to capture help-seeking attitudes for themselves as well as for their child. The GHSQ has been shown to have acceptable to good internal consistency (α = .70-.85) and good test-retest reliability (r = .85-.92) (Hammer & Spiker, 2018; Wilson et al., 2005).

Table 2

Measurement Details and Internal Consistencies for the Study Sample

Measure Name	Number of Items (*n*)	Cronbach's α
Public Stigma	15 items (*n=250*)	.86
Devaluation of Consumers Who Have Serious Mental Illness	8 items (*n=250*)	.83
Devaluation of Families of Consumers Who Have Serious Mental Illness	7 items (*n=250*)	.69
Parents' Self-Stigma Scale	11 items (*n=250*)	.83
Vicarious Stigma Scale	12 items (*n=165*)	.95
Sad	6 items (*n=171*)	.94
Angry	6 items (*n=169*)	.90
The Center for Epidemiological Studies Short Depression Scale	10 items (*n=250*)	.67
The General Help-Seeking Questionnaire	22 items (*n=164*)	.84
Parent	11 items (*n=179*)	.81
Child	11 items (*n=187*)	.71

Note. Variations in *n* due to "not applicable" option for scale items.

3.6   Statistical Analyses

Descriptive statistics of estimated means, frequencies, and standard deviations of all measures are included in the study. Pearson product-moment correlations are used to estimate associations between public stigma, self-stigma, vicarious stigma, depression, and help-seeking. Analyses to check distributions were used to assess normality of data. Descriptive and correlation analyses have been conducted using SPSS v. 23 (IBM Corp., 2015).

Completion time, IP address frequencies, consistent answers to demographic questions, and the attention check question were utilized to identify participants with low quality data to be excluded. Using the "forced choice" option in Qualtrics minimized the amount of missing data. Some items allow for an "n/a" or "prefer not to answer" option, which will not be treated as missing. Three of the measures included in this study, The Vicarious Stigma Scale and The General Help-Seeking Questionnaire (parent/caregiver and child), allow for an "n/a" option, which will not be treated as missing. All scale scores will be computed by calculating the mean of items, this way, scale scores will only include items that are relevant to the participant's life as well as reducing the amount of excluded cases when the n/a option is selected. For instance, The Vicarious Stigma Scale asks participants how sad they would be if their child was not selected for a sport's team due to their mental health challenges, but not all children participate in sports. Therefore, it would be most accurate for a participant in this situation to select "n/a" for this item.

A confirmatory factor analysis (CFA) was conducted for The Vicarious Stigma Scale in order to further examine the 2-factor structure of sadness and anger of this newly created measure. The following fit indices used in this study include chi-squared, standardized root mean square residual (SMAR), root mean square error of approximation (RMSEA), Tucker-Lewis index (TLI), and comparative fit index (CFI) (Brown & Moore, 2012; Hu & Bentler, 1999). The following fit guidelines were utilized to assess model fit – a non-significant chi-squared; SMAR less than 0.08; RMSEA less than 0.06; TLI greater than 0.95; CFI greater than 0.95. Together, these fit indices provide a reliable and conservative approach to evaluating the model. The CFA analysis was conducted utilizing an opensource statistical software jamovi and relevant packages

(Epskamp et al., 2017; R Core Team, 2021; Rosseel et al., 2018; The jamovi project, 2022).

Hypotheses were tested with path analysis within a structural equation modeling framework. Fit indices were examined to evaluate the model fit, which include Chi-Square, Root Mean Square of Approximation (RMSEA), Goodness of Fit Index (GFI), Standard Mean Square Residual (SRMR), Non-Normed Fit Index (NNFI; also known as the Tucker-Lewis Index), and Comparative Fit Index (CFI). The following criteria for goodness of fit for each statistic are as follows – Chi-Square $p > .05$; RMSEA ≤ 0.07; GFI ≥ 0.95; SRMR ≤ 0.8; NNFI ≥ 0.95; CFI ≥ 0.95 (Hooper, Coughlan & Mullen, 2008). Modification indices were also utilized to explore alternative paths in order to determine best model fit. Betas were examined for each path in the model for significance, which examined the hypothesized relationships within the proposed model. Path analyses utilized the opensource statistical software RStudio and relevant packages (Epskamp et al., 2017; Pornprasertmanit et al., 2021; Rosseel et al., 2018; RStudio Team, 2022).

An a priori power analysis of norms was examined in order to identify a sufficient sample size for the study. Kline (2015) suggests recruiting approximately 10-20 participants for each parameter in a mediation model. The presented model contains 2 exogenous factors, 5 endogenous factors, and 5 error terms. The presented model contains 7 direct paths and 5 indirect paths. Parameters can be calculated by finding the sum of error terms, direct paths, and indirect paths; this equals 17 parameters for the presented model. Thus, suggesting a sample size of 170-340. To account for quality of data, a sample size of 250 participants was collected for this study.

CHAPTER 4

RESULTS

4.1   Quantitative Investigation

A total of 760 individuals participated in the pre-screener survey, which indicated 259 eligible participants for the main dissertation survey (Figure 6). The current investigation has a total sample size of 250 participants. All participants in the final sample answered the attention check question correctly, were found to have consistent answers to demographic questions, and answered all survey questions presented.

Figure 6

Prisma Diagram for Quantitative Investigation

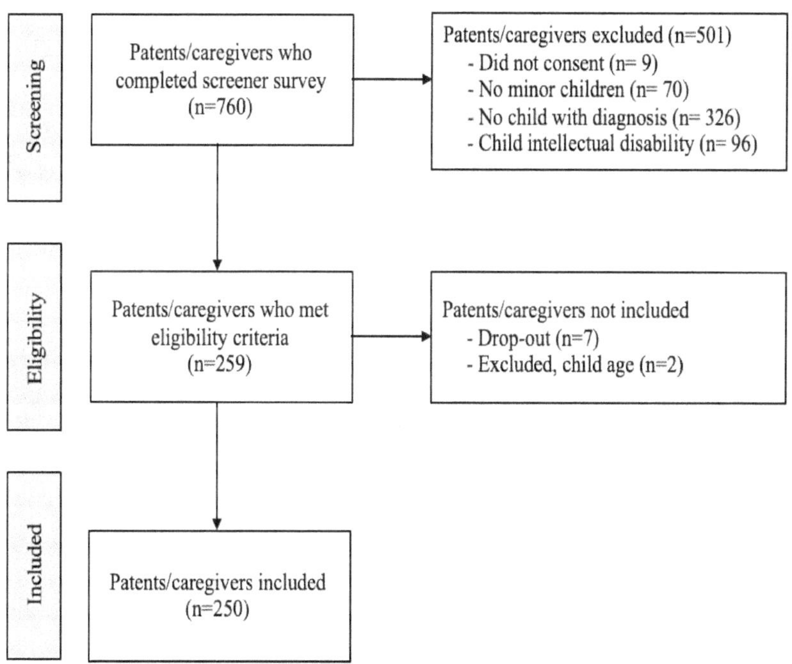

Using the "forced choice" option in Qualtrics and utilizing scale means minimized the amount of missing data, however, three scales allowed participants to select "n/a" for items that were not relevant to their lives. Items on the measures of help-seeking and vicarious stigma were analyzed and particular cases were examined further for quality. Among the three scales, a total of 129 cases (51.6%) in this sample had at least one missing data point and 6.04% of scale items were missing.

All participant scale scores were able to be calculated for both help-seeking measures and were used in all analyses using these variables. A total of 71 cases (28.4%) in the sample had at least one missing data point on the measure of help-seeking for parents/caregivers and 3.86% of scale items were missing. When answering items about the likelihood of seeking support for themselves, the items that received the most n/a responses included seeking support from their child's teacher (15.2%), "I would not seek help" (7.6%), and seeking help from their partner (6%). A total of 63 cases (25.2%) in the sample had at least one missing data point on the measure of help-seeking for their child and 2.98% of scale items were missing. When answering items about the likelihood of seeking support for their child, the items that received the most n/a responses included "I would not seek help" (10.8%) and seeking help from their partner (7.2%).

Of the participants who responded n/a to the item stating "I would not seek help," this was the only item that n/a was selected on that help-seeking scale for the majority of participants (78.95% of participants regarding help-seeking for themselves; 74.07% regarding help-seeking for their child). Of note, all participants who responded n/a to seeking support for themselves from their partner also responded n/a to seeking support for their child from this source (n=15). However, there were three participants who only responded n/a to seeking support for their child from their partner, and all three of these participants did not select n/a for any other items on the scale regarding help-seeking for their child.

A total of 79 cases (31.6%) in the sample had at least one missing data point on the measure of vicarious stigma and 15.67% of scale items were missing. When asked about the sadness related to witnessing the stigmatization of their child, the items that received the most n/a responses included relatives excluding their child from family functions (22.4%) and their child not being chosen to be part of a sport's team (18.8%) due to their mental health challenges.

A total of 8 cases (3.2%) in the sample were excluded from some analyses due to answering n/a to all items on the vicarious stigma sad scale. The majority of these 8 participants answered all other survey questions. Two of these 8 participants endorsed n/a on one additional item – both participants responded n/a to seeking support for themselves from their child's teacher. Therefore, these participants will not be excluded for analyses of other variables of interest. Sample size will be noted when impacted by these cases. Therefore, analyses using the full scale will have a sample of 250 or 242 depending on the variables that are included.

Analyses to check distributions were used to assess normality of data. The skewness of measure scores ranged from .07 to .78 and kurtosis ranged from .07 to .44, which are within acceptable limits. Thus, variable data was not transformed to yield a normal distribution.

4.2 Descriptive Analyses

The demographic characteristics for the parent/caregiver-participants are presented in Table 3. Results showed that of the 250 participants, the mean age was 37.05 (SD=8.48); and the majority of the sample identified as female (73.2%, n=183) and white (72%, n=180). Participants were located around the world representing 21 different countries, including the United Kingdom (30.4%, n=76), South Africa (20.8%, n=52), the United States (18.8%, n=47), and Canada (11.2%, n=28). The majority of participants also endorsed experiencing their own mental health challenges (58%, n=145) and endorsed receiving some type of treatment for their mental health challenges (58.4%, n=146). The most commonly reported parental mental health challenges include depression, anxiety, ADHD, and PTSD.

Parents/caregivers also answered survey questions specifically about their child with mental health challenges, and if they have more than one child with mental health challenges, they were either prompted to report on the child with the most recent birthday or they were contacted by the researcher to determine which child to think about when answering questions. The majority of participants reported having 1 minor child with mental health challenges (90%, n=225), and the majority of participants reported being that child's biological parent (92.8%, n=232).

Table 3

Parent/Caregiver Demographics

Variable	% (N) or M (SD)
Age	37.05 (8.48)
Gender	
Female	73.2% (183)
Male	26.4% (66)
Non-binary	.4% (1)
Race	
White	72% (180)
African American, Black	22% (55)
Middle Eastern	2.4% (6)
Asian	1.6% (4)
Prefer not to specify	2% (5)
Ethnicity	
Hispanic/Latinx	8.8% (22)
Not Hispanic/Latinx	82.8% (207)
Prefer not to specify	8.4% (21)
Caregiver Diagnosed with Mental Health Challenges	
Yes	58% (145)
No	42% (105)
Indicated Caregiver Mental Health Challenges	
Depression	28.9% (72)
Anxiety	27.7% (69)
Attention-Deficit/Hyperactivity Disorder	7.6% (19)
Post-Traumatic Stress Disorder	5.6% (14)
Obsessive-Compulsive Disorder	2% (5)
Autism Spectrum Disorder	.8% (2)
Bipolar Disorder	.8% (2)
Prefer not to specify	8.4% (21)

Variable	% (N) or M (SD)
Treatments/Supports Received for Caregiver Mental Health Challenges	
Individual Therapy/Counseling	45.2% (113)
Medication	41.2% (103)
Group Therapy	6.4% (16)
Support Group	6% (15)
Other	1.2% (3)
Prefer not to specify	.8% (2)
No Treatment	41% (102)
Marital Status	
Married	58.4% (146)
Single	26.4% (66)
Common Law	9.6% (24)
Divorced	5.6% (14)
Education Level	
Some High School	2% (5)
High School Degree	9.6% (24)
Some College	16.4% (41)
College Degree	31.2% (78)
Some Graduate School	6.8% (17)
Graduate Degree	34% (85)
Employment Status	
Full-time	57.6% (144)
Part-time	27.2% (68)
Not employed	13.6% (34)
Prefer not to specify	1.6% (4)
Yearly Family Income (USD)	
$0-$25,000	22.4% (56)
$25,001-$49,999	26.4% (66)
$50,000-$74,999	18.4% (46)
$75,000-$99,999	18% (45)
$100,000-$149,000	9.6% (24)
>$150,000	4.4% (11)
Prefer not to specify	.8% (2)

Variable	% (N) or M (SD)
Caregiver's Total Minor Children with Mental Health Diagnosis	
1 Child	90% (225)
2 Children	8.4% (21)
3 Children	1.2% (3)
4 Children	.4% (1)
Caregiver Relationship to their Child with Mental Health Diagnosis	
Biological Parent	92.8% (232)
Step-Parent	3.2% (8)
Foster Parent	2.4% (6)
Other	1.6% (4)
Country of Residence	
United Kingdom	30.4% (76)
South Africa	20.8% (52)
United States	18.8% (47)
Canada	11.2% (28)
Mexico	4% (10)
Poland	3.2% (8)
Ireland	1.6% (4)
Netherlands	1.6% (4)
Portugal	1.6% (4)
Spain	1.2% (3)
Belgium	.8% (2)
Hungary	.8% (2)
New Zealand	.8% (2)
Chile	.4% (1)
Czech Republic	.4% (1)
Denmark	.4% (1)
Israel	.4% (1)
Italy	.4% (1)
Norway	.4% (1)
Sweden	.4% (1)
Switzerland	.4% (1)

N=250

Child reported demographics can be found in Table 4. Results showed that of the 250 identified children, the mean age was 9.34 years-old (*SD*=4.47); and the majority of participants identified their child as male (58%, n=145). The most commonly reported child mental health diagnoses in this sample include anxiety, ADHD, autism spectrum disorder, behavior problem in child, and depression. The mean age the child received their primary diagnosis was 7 years-old (*SD*=3.85). The majority of parents/caregivers reported that their child's pediatrician/general practitioner/other MD provided the primary diagnosis (54.8%, n=137). A "check all that apply" option was presented regarding treatments/supports received by the child; the majority of participants endorsed at least 1 type of treatment (e.g., individual therapy, school accommodations/services, medication), a small number of participants reported that their child is not currently receiving treatment/supports for their mental health challenges (1.2%, n=3).

Table 4

Child Demographics

Variable	% (N) or M (SD)
Age	
	9.34 (4.47)
Gender	
Male	58% (145)
Female	40.8% (102)
Non-binary	1.2% (3)
Race	
White	70.8% (177)
African American, Black	23.6% (59)
Middle Eastern	2% (5)
Asian	1.2% (3)
American Indian, Alaskan Native	.4% (1)
Prefer not to specify	2% (5)

Variable	% (N) or M (SD)
Ethnicity	
Hispanic/Latinx	9.2% (23)
Not Hispanic/Latinx	83.2% (208)
Prefer not to specify	7.6% (19)
Age Received Primary Mental Health Diagnosis	7.00 (3.85)
Primary Diagnosed Mental Health Challenge	
Anxiety	30.8% (77)
Attention-Deficit/Hyperactivity Disorder	28% (70)
Autism Spectrum Disorder	21.2% (53)
Behavior problem in child	7.2% (18)
Depression	4.4% (11)
Post-Traumatic Stress Disorder	1.6% (4)
Oppositional-Defiant Disorder	1.2% (3)
Obsessive-Compulsive Disorder	.8% (2)
Adjustment disorder	.4% (1)
Bipolar Disorder	.4% (1)
Conduct Disorder	.4% (1)
Selective mutism	.4% (1)
Global Developmental Delay	.4% (1)
Other	1.6% (4)
Prefer not to specify	1.2% (3)
Primary Mental Health Diagnosis Provided By	
Pediatrician, GP, other MD	54.8% (137)
Psychologist	32.4% (81)
Psychiatrist	8% (20)
School Professional	2.4% (6)
Other	1.6% (4)
Prefer not to specify	.8% (2)
Treatments/Supports Received	
Individual Therapy	52.6% (131)
School Accommodations & Services	35.7% (89)
Family Therapy	24.9% (62)
Medication	24.8% (62)
Parenting Classes	16.5% (41)
IEP	10.8% (27)
Other	5.6% (14)
Prefer not to specify	3.2% (8)
No treatment	1.2% (3)

Variable	% (N) or M (SD)
All Diagnosed Mental Health Challenges	
Anxiety	46.6% (116)
Attention-Deficit/Hyperactivity Disorder	34.8% (87)
Autism Spectrum Disorder	22.5% (56)
Behavior problem in child	13.3% (33)
Depression	10.8% (27)
Post-Traumatic Stress Disorder	4% (10)
Obsessive-Compulsive Disorder	3.2% (8)
Oppositional-Defiant Disorder	2.4% (6)
Adjustment disorder	2.4% (6)
Bipolar Disorder	2.4% (6)
Conduct Disorder	1.2% (3)
Selective mutism	1.6% (4)
Global Developmental Delay	.8% (2)
Other	4.4% (11)
Prefer not to specify	1.2% (3)

N=250

4.3   Confirmatory Factor Analysis

Prior work examined this The Vicarious Stigma Scale utilizing an exploratory factor analysis (EFA) with a Varimax rotation (Serchuk et al., 2021). The results of the EFA indicated a 2-factor solution, labeled as Vicarious Stigma Sad and Vicarious Stigma Angry, each consisting of 6-items. To further examine this measure, a confirmatory factor analysis (CFA) was conducted for the Vicarious Stigma Scale based on the data collected in this study. Based on the previous findings, the estimated model included 2 factors (sad and angry) and 6 indicators each (Figure 7).

Figure 7

Vicarious Stigma Scale CFA Model and Standardized Loadings (Standardized Errors)

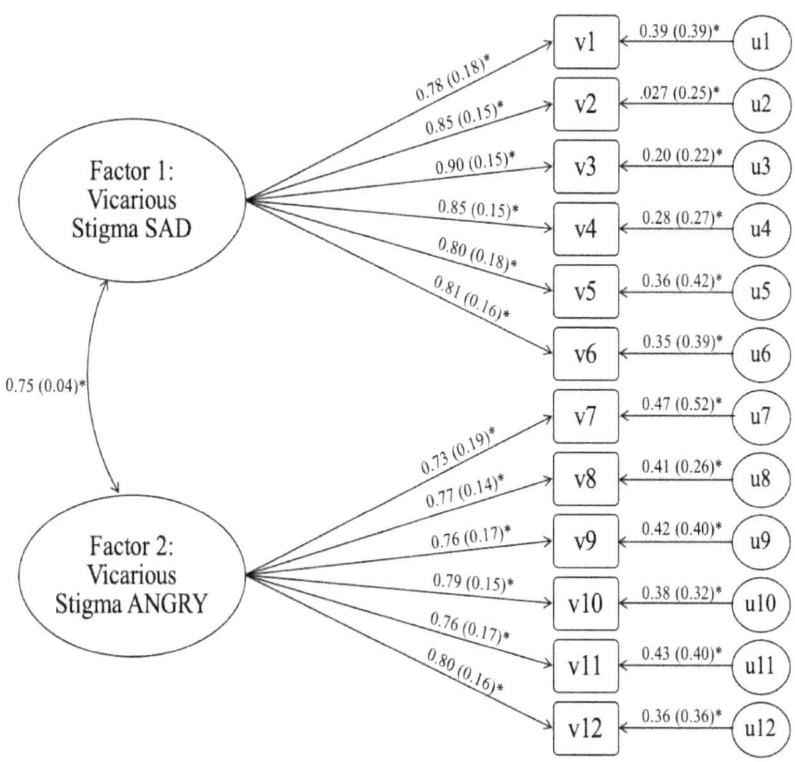

Note. N=165
*$p < 0.001$

Although all paths were significant (p<0.001; Figure 8), the model achieved poor fit, $\chi^2(53)$ = 409, SMAR = 0.07, RMSEA = 0.17 (CI = 0.15 to 0.18); TLI = 0.78, CFI = 0.83. Fit was achieved regarding the non-significant chi-squared and SMNAR statistic, however, the three other indices did not fall within the range of fit. To further examine this measure, additional CFA's were conducted. This measure asks participants the same set of questions across the two dimensions of sad and angry. Based on the scale content and the significant paths for each factor above, the following estimated models each included 1 factor with 6 indicators (Figure 8; Figure 9).

Figure 8

Vicarious Stigma - Sad CFA Model and Standardized Loadings (Standardized Errors)

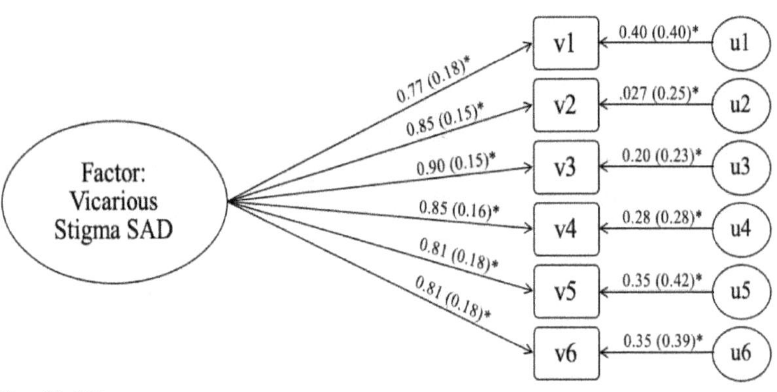

Note. N=171

*p<0.001

Figure 9

Vicarious Stigma - Angry CFA Model and Standardized Loadings (Standardized Errors)

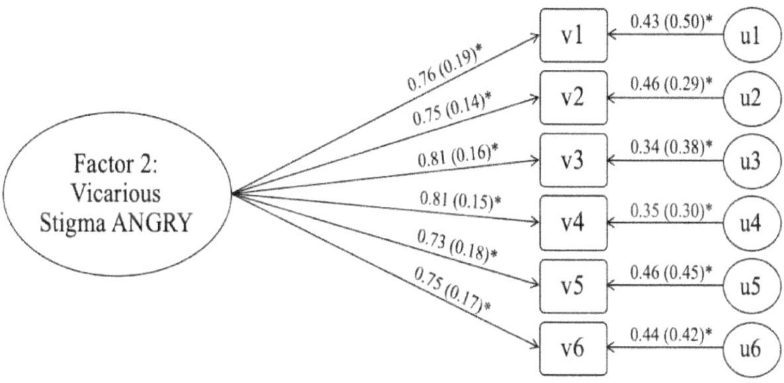

Note. N=169

**p<0.001*

The one-factor model examining vicarious stigma sadness with 6 indicators achieved fit (Figure 8), $\chi^2(9) = 33.5$, SMAR = 0.03, RMSEA = 0.11 (CI = 0.06 to 0.15); TLI = 0.96, CFI = 0.97. Although the RMSEA statistic for this model did not fall within the fit guidelines, all other indices did achieve fit according to the guidelines for the vicarious stigma sad CFA. The one-factor model examining vicarious stigma anger with 6 indicators did not achieve fit (Figure 9), $\chi^2(9) = 115$, SMAR = 0.07, RMSEA = 0.22 (CI = 0.19 to 0.26); TLI = 0.76, CFI = 0.86. Similar to the original CFA, only two of the indices (chi-squared and SMAR) were within the range of fit for the vicarious stigma angry CFA. Therefore, vicarious stigma angry will be excluded from analyses. Vicarious stigma sad will be utilized in the following analyses.

4.4   Correlation Analyses

Pearson correlation analyses of the study sample, related to hypotheses 1-6, are presented in Table 5. In the total sample, public stigma towards parents/caregivers of children with mental health challenges showed significant positive relation with self-stigma ($r = .28$, $p < .001$) and depression ($r = .30$, $p < .001$). Thus, supporting hypotheses 1. Demonstrating partial support for hypothesis 2, public stigma towards individuals with mental health challenges had a significant positive relation with depression ($r = .21$, $p < .001$). Self-stigma was found to have a significant positive relation with public stigma towards individuals with mental health challenges ($r = .15$, $p < .05$), vicarious stigma sad ($r = .22$, $p < .001$) and depression ($r = .32$, $p < .001$), and a significant negative relation with help-seeking for themselves ($r = -.17$, $p < .01$). Thus, supporting hypothesis 4, and demonstrating partial support for hypothesis 5. Vicarious stigma sad was found to have a significant positive relation with depression ($r = .16$, $p < .01$) and help-seeking for their child ($r = .13$, $p < .05$). Thus, demonstrating support for hypothesis 6. The analyses did not demonstrate support for hypothesis 3, where public stigma towards parents/caregivers did not have a significant relation to either of the help-seeking variables.

Table 5

Sample Correlations, Means, Standard Deviations, and Ranges for Study Variables

	1	2	3	4	5	6	7
1. Public Stigma Customers	-						
2. Public Stigma Parents/Caregivers	.62***	-					
3. Self-Stigma	.15*	.28***	-				
4. Vicarious Stigma Sad[a]	.10	.10	.22***	-			
5. Depression	.21***	.30***	.32***	.16**	-		
6. Help-Seeking for Parent/Caregiver	.08	-.05	-.17**	-.002	-.04	-	
7. Help-Seeking for Child	.06	.05	.01	.13*	.01	.48***	-
Mean	2.54	2.61	2.19	7.21	2.30	4.31	5.10
Standard Deviation	.51	.45	.64	2.56	.45	1.09	.93
Range	2.75	2.29	3.64	9.00	2.30	5.82	5.20

[a] n=242
*p < .05, **p < .01, ***p < .001

4.5   Path Analyses

As discussed, this study proposed to examine the role of public, self- and vicarious stigma in relation to symptoms of depression and help-seeking. Results of the originally proposed path model (Figure 1) can be found below (Figure 10). The overall model fit was poor, $\chi^2(10) = 29.22$, RMSEA = 0.09, GFI = 0.96, SRMR = 0.07, NNFI = 0.71, CFI = 0.86.

Figure 10

Hypothesized Path Model

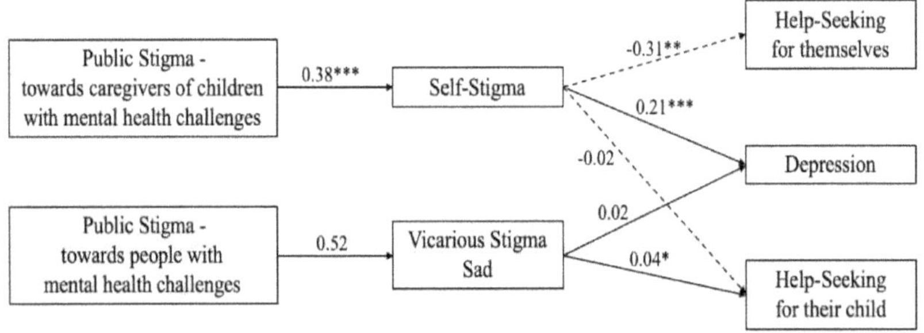

Note. N=242

*p < 0.05, **p < 0.005**, ***p < 0.001.

Due to the poor fit of the original hypothesized model, additional analyses were conducted. The hypothesized model was split into 2 different path models that were tested – the first focusing on self-stigma and the second vicarious stigma sad.

4.6.1   Self-Stigma Path Models. The following path model examines the role of public stigma towards caregivers and self-stigma in relation to symptoms of depression and help-seeking (Figure 11). The overall model fit did not meet criteria, $\chi^2(3) = 14.72$, RMSEA = 0.13, GFI = 0.97, SRMR = 0.06, NNFI = 0.70, CFI = 0.91.

Figure 11

Self-Stigma Path Model

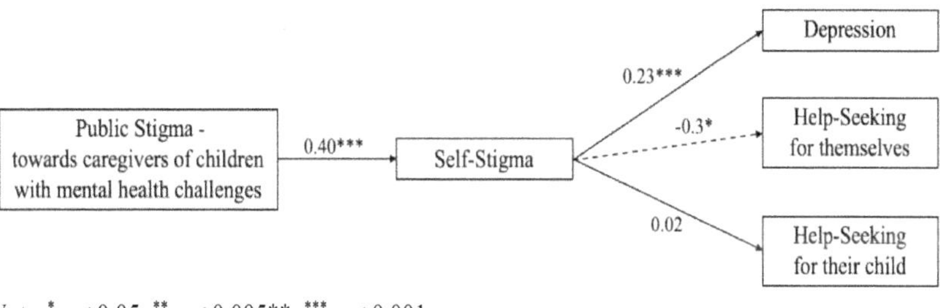

Note. * p < 0.05, ** p < 0.005**, *** p < 0.001.

Due to poor fit of the model above (Figure 11), modification indices were utilized. The strongest relationship was public stigma towards caregivers and depression (MI=13.59). Hence, an additional path between public stigma and depression was added to the model. The results from this next path model can be found below (Figure 12).

Figure 12

Self-Stigma Path Model with Partial Mediation

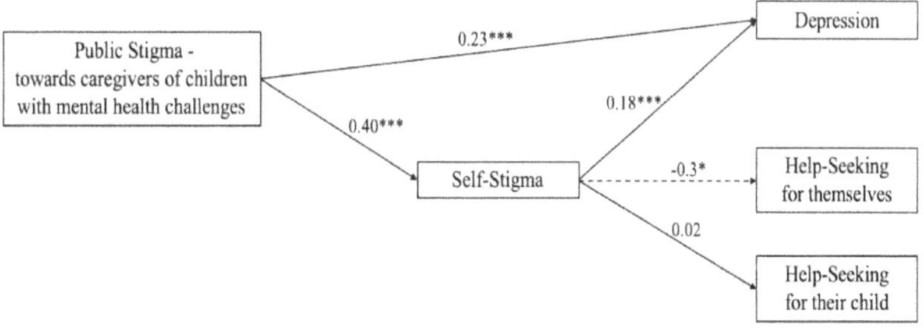

Note. * p < 0.05, ** p < 0.005**, *** p < 0.001.

The overall model fit was excellent, $\chi^2(2) = 0.70$, RMSEA < 0.001, GFI = 1.00, SRMR = 0.01, NNFI = 1.05, CFI = 1.00 (Figure 12). The majority of paths were significant. Self-stigma did not significantly predict help-seeking for their child. Public stigma towards caregivers was positively associated with self-stigma and depression. Self-stigma was positively associated with depression and negatively associated with help-seeking for themselves. The relationship between public stigma towards parents/caregivers, help-seeking for themselves, and depression was mediated by self-stigma. Thus, providing additional support for hypotheses 1 and 4, and demonstrating partial support for hypotheses 5 and 7.

4.6.2   Vicarious Stigma Path Models. The second path model that was tested examines the role of public stigma towards people with mental health challenges and vicarious stigma in relation to symptoms of depression and help-seeking for their child (Figure 13). The overall model fit did not meet criteria, $\chi^2(2) = 8.64$, RMSEA = 0.12, GFI = 0.98, SRMR = 0.06, NNFI = -0.27, CFI = 0.58.

Figure 13

Vicarious Stigma Sad Path Model

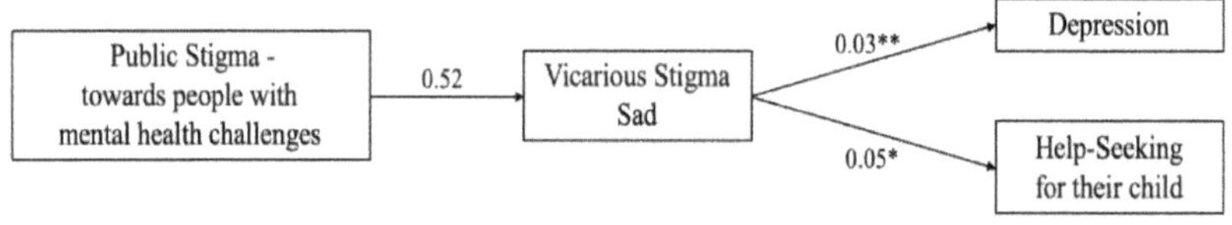

Note. N=242

*p < 0.05, ** p < 0.005**, *** p < 0.001.

Due to poor fit of the model above (Figure 13), modification indices were utilized. The strongest relationship was public stigma towards people with mental health challenges and depression (MI=8.47). Hence, an additional path between public stigma and depression was added to the model. The results from this path model can be found below (Figure 14).

Figure 14

Vicarious Stigma Sad Path Model with Partial Mediation

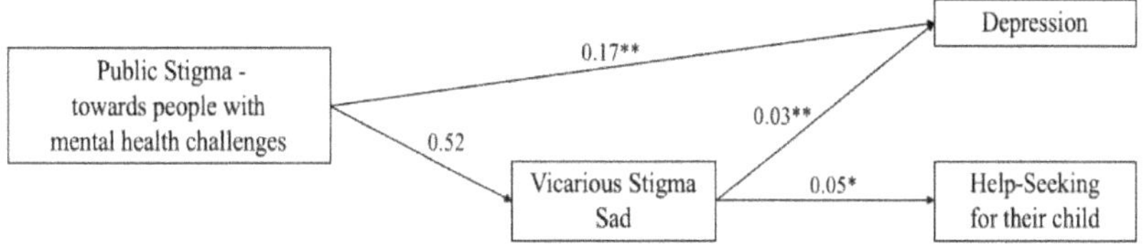

Note. N=242

*p < 0.05, **p < 0.005**, ***p < 0.001.

The overall model fit was excellent, $\chi^2(1) = 0.02$, RMSEA < 0.001, GFI = 1.00, SRMR = 0.003, NNFI = 1.38, CFI = 1.00 (Figure 14). The majority of paths were significant. Public stigma towards people with mental health challenges did not significantly predict vicarious stigma sad. Public stigma towards people with mental health challenges was positively associated with depression. Vicarious stigma sad was positively associated with depression and help-seeking for their child. Thus, providing additional support for hypothesis 6, and partial support for hypotheses 2 and 8.

CHAPTER 5

DISCUSSION

The present study aimed to examine differential associations with self-stigma and vicarious stigma on parents/caregivers of children with mental health challenges. Additionally, this study examined a novel measure of vicarious stigma. Consistent with previous research (e.g., Chan & Leung, 2021), results indicated that stigma was an important aspect of the parents'/caregivers' experiences regarding depression symptoms and attitudes towards help-seeking.

The Vicarious Stigma Scale is a novel measure that utilized community-based participatory research for item development, and a confirmatory factor analysis (CFA) was conducted with this sample to further understand the structure of this measure. Prior work examining The Vicarious Stigma Scale conducted an exploratory factor analysis (EFA) with a Varimax rotation, which indicated a 2-factor solution, labeled as Vicarious Stigma Sad and Vicarious Stigma Angry, each consisting of 6-items (Serchuk et al., 2021). The CFA conducted as part of the current investigation found that the 2-factor model provides a poor fit according to widely accepted fit indices guidelines (Brown & Moore, 2012; Hu & Bentler, 1999). Additional CFA's were conducted utilizing a 1-factor solutions consisting of 6-items each (e.g., one with only items related to sadness, one with only items related to anger). Results of the CFA supported a 1-factor solution, which only includes items related to sadness. The sadness dimension of The Vicarious Stigma Scale is consistent with the limited amount of previous literature discussing aspects of vicarious stigma experienced by parents of children with mental health challenges (e.g., Chan & Leung, 2021; Eaton et al., 2016). For instance, in a study utilizing semi-structured interviews with parents of minor children with mental health challenges, Eaton, Ohan, Strizke, and Corrigan (2016) found that parents who experienced the stigmatization of their child vicariously reported feelings of sadness, frustration, helplessness, and guilt. Excluding the previous study first examining the Vicarious Stigma Scale, to the writer's knowledge, there has not been any literature examining anger in relation to parent/caregiver experiences of vicarious stigma.

All of the predicted relations among the types of stigma examined and depression were supported. Correlation analyses indicated that higher levels of reported public stigma, self-stigma, and vicarious stigma were all found to be related to experiencing greater depression symptoms. These findings are consistent with previous literature discussing the associations between the experiences of public stigma, self-stigma, and vicarious stigma with symptoms of depression such as sadness and feelings of guilt in parents/caregivers of children with mental health challenges (e.g., Chen et al., 2021; Eaton et al., 2020; Mickelson, 2001). Following the demanding and distressing nature of being a parent experiencing stigma, these findings add to the current literature on the experiences of stigma by parents/caregivers of children with mental health challenges. Future research investigating the specific nature of the types of stigmas in relation to the emotional impacts may help to better understand the effects of stigma in this population.

Some of predicted relations among types of help-seeking behaviors and stigma were supported. Correlation analyses indicated that higher levels of parent-/caregiver-reported self-stigma were found to be related to having less favorable attitudes towards help-seeking for themselves. This finding is consistent with related previous literature, where parents of children with mental health challenges who reported experiencing higher levels of self-stigma was related to negative attitudes towards help-seeking (e.g., Conceição, Rothes, & Gusmão, 2021). Further, the current cross-sectional investigation found self-stigma to be a significant mediator between public stigma towards parents/caregivers of children with mental health challenges, and help-seeking for themselves and depression via path analysis. In other words, higher levels of public stigma towards parents/caregivers and higher levels of self-stigma were related to less favorable attitudes towards help-seeking for themselves and more depression symptoms endorsed. These findings are consistent with previous literature finding self-stigma to be a significant mediator between public stigma and help-seeking attitudes in a population of individuals with mental health challenges (e.g., Vogel, Wade, & Hackler, 2007). These finding further support the idea that parents/caregivers of children with mental health challenges experiencing self-stigma endorse common public beliefs of blame and/or incompetence, and in turn, respond by avoiding or delaying engagement in help-seeking behaviors (Corrigan, 2004; Zisman-Ilani et al., 2013).

As predicted, correlation analyses indicated that higher levels of parent-/caregiver-reported vicarious stigma were related to more favorable attitudes towards help-seeking for their child with mental health challenges. Although these specific variables have not been examined in the existing literature to this date, this finding is consistent with literature examining different responses to stigma such as "righteous indignation" – where individuals recognize the injustice of stigma and experience feelings of personal empowerment (Corrigan & Rao, 2012). Further, the current cross-sectional investigation found vicarious stigma to be a significant mediator between public stigma towards people with mental health challenges, and help-seeking for their child and depression via path analysis. In other words, higher levels of public stigma towards people with mental health challenges and higher levels of self-stigma were related to more favorable attitudes towards help-seeking for their child and more depression symptoms endorsed.

Public stigma towards parents/caregivers of children with mental health challenges was not found to have a significant relation with help-seeking for themselves or for their child. More research is needed to better understand the specifics regarding parent/caregiver experiences of public stigma and how it related to help-seeking behaviors and attitudes. Further, parent/caregiver self-stigma was not found to have a significant relation with help-seeking for their child with mental health. This finding is supported by research, which found that self-stigma did not affect parent's attitudes to engage in help-seeking related to their child (Dempster et al., 2013).

5.1   Limitations

There are several limitations of this study. There are limitations regarding the lack of diversity in this sample in terms of the parents/caregivers as well as their children. Specifically, in terms of the parents/caregivers, descriptive statistics indicated homogeneity in gender identity, race, ethnicity, relationship to child (e.g., biological parent), and the number of minor children who have received a mental health diagnosis. These aspects of the sample may limit the generalizability of results. Future research examining the experiences of stigma by parents/caregivers of children with mental health challenges should aim to obtain a more diverse sample regarding characteristics of the parents/caregivers as well as their children in order to more comprehensively understand experiences of stigma in this population.

Limitations exist regarding interpreting results related to attitudes towards help-seeking in this sample of participants. Approximately half of parent-/caregiver-participants indicated having a mental health diagnosis (58%), receiving treatment/supports for themselves (59%), and the majority of participant's children have received at treatment/support (95.6%). According to SAMHSA, the 2021 National Survey on Drug Use and Health, an average of 22.8% of adults in the United States report having a mental health diagnosis and an average of 47.2% of these adults have received mental health services within the past year (2022). In an international sample, The World Health Organization reports prevalence rates of adults with a mental health diagnosis to range from 10.9% to 15.6% (2022). According to the Child and Adolescent Health Measurement Initiative, 2016-2019 National Surveys of Children's Health, an average of 10.1% of children and adolescents (ages 3-17) in the United States received treatment from a mental health professional within the past year according to parent-report (Bitsko et al., 2022). In summary, this sample had a higher prevalence of adult mental health challenges than the general public as well as higher levels of reported engagement in treatments/supports for themselves and for their child's mental health challenges.

Several factors may relate to the high prevalence of reported help-seeking behaviors in the current sample, one of which may be related to participants' race/ethnicity. While stigma has generally been found to deter individuals from help-seeking, research has found this relation to be stronger for racial/ethnic minorities (Clement et al., 2015; Maura & Weisman de Mamani, 2017; Misra, Jackson, Chong, Choe, Tay, Wong, & Yang, 2021). Structural stigma, public stigma from family members, public stigma related to lack of knowledge and cultural beliefs, and self-stigma were identified by Misra and colleagues (2021) as noteworthy barriers to help-seeking in a systematic review examining cultural factors related to stigma and mental illness among Black, Asian, and Latinx Americans. The participants in the current study consisted predominantly of White participants (72% of parents/caregivers; 70.8% of their identified children), who may have faced fewer social and environmental barriers, and thus, report higher than average help-seeking behaviors for themselves and their child compared to the general public. Therefore, there is a limited scope of exploration of racial-/ethnicity-based factors contributing to these outcomes. Given these issues, generalizability of this study on help-seeking may be limited. Future investigations should examine the relationship between current help-seeking and willingness to seek help in a more diverse sample. Further, research is needed to comprehensively examine aspects of power structures as a means of creating and perpetuating stigma related to culture and help-seeking as well as culturally-informed stigma reduction strategies (Misra et al., 2021).

Limitations exist regarding the measures utilized in this study. The current investigation utilized a measure of public stigma that asked participants about stigma towards individuals in general with mental health challenges, rather than specifying stigma towards children. Although the public stigma measure was already adapted for the purposes of this study, additionally changing the questions to specifically ask about children would have made the questions more relevant to this study. Additionally, the current investigation utilized the relatively novel measure of vicarious stigma, thus, there is limited psychometric testing. In the current study, The Vicarious Stigma Scale had participants answer questions related to the sadness and anger they felt in various situations where their child is stigmatized. This investigation found some support for the sad emotional response of vicarious stigma using this measure, however, did not find support for the angry emotional response. Using the two specific emotional reactions of sadness and anger may have been a drawback of examining vicarious stigma in this study. It is possible that other emotional experiences (e.g., feeling guilty, anxious) or using a more general term (e.g., feeling negative emotions) may better capture the emotional response of vicarious stigma experiences by parents/caregivers of children with mental health challenges. Future studies should utilize community based participatory research to better understand the emotional experiences of the population of parents/caregivers of children with mental health challenges when facing vicarious stigma. Further research is needed examining the Vicarious Stigma Scale as well as the construct of vicarious stigma in a population of parents/caregivers of children with mental health challenges.

5.2   Strengths, Implications, and Future Directions

This study has several strengths and the findings of this investigation add to the small body of literature devoted to examining stigma experienced parents/caregivers of children with mental health challenges. The use of qualitative interviews with stakeholders to inform recruitment materials and adaptations to measures is a significant strength of this study. It is important for researchers to amplify the voices of people with lived experience when investigating specific populations, thus allowing for more authentic and representative information to be obtained as well as disseminated. Future studies should continue to engage individuals with lived experience from populations of interest in various aspects of the research process.

Although limitations have been noted regarding a lack of diversity in important demographic variables related to the parents/caregivers and their children, there are strengths regarding the sample collected. Utilizing online crowdsourcing for participant recruitment, a sample of participants representing 21 different countries was collected. Previous research examining stigma experiences of parents/caregivers of children with mental health challenges have typically recruited participants from a particular country/region. Experiences of stigma are known to be intertwined with culture. A significant strength of the current investigation was replicating findings related to stigma variables as well as depression and help-seeking in an international sample. Although many countries were represented by participants in this sample, the majority of participants were from 4 countries (81.2%) – United Kingdom, South Africa, United States, and Canada. More research is needed to examine the impacts and experiences of stigma on parents/caregivers in an international sample.

Another strength of this study includes replicating findings regarding the relation of self-stigma with depression and help-seeking in a population of parents/caregivers of children with mental health challenges. Specifically, higher levels of self-stigma were related to less favorable attitudes towards help-seeking for themselves, and was not significantly associated with attitudes towards help-seeking for their child. There is a need to more comprehensively understand these variables within this population of parents/caregivers. Differentiating measurement of attitudes towards help-seeking for themselves and their child is another strength of this study. More research is needed to understand how stigma is associated with different forms of seeking support in this population. Further, replicating the relation of vicarious stigma with depression adds to the tiny body of literature examining this novel aspect of stigma. Successfully replicating results related to variables of interest created a good opportunity to examine vicarious stigma in this population as well as the relation of vicarious stigma with help-seeking. This is the first study to the writer's knowledge examining vicarious stigma related to help-seeking in a population of parents/caregivers of children with mental health challenges. Higher levels of vicarious stigma was found to be related to more favorable attitudes towards help-seeking for their child. Providing data to begin addressing this identified gap in the literature is a significant strength of the current investigation. Future studies should continue to investigate the differential relation of self-stigma and vicarious stigma with help-seeking variables.

The current investigation provides a snap-shot into stigma experiences of parents/caregivers of children with mental health challenges. Future studies should investigate stigma experiences longitudinally to see how these variables effect this specific population over time. For instance, it may be helpful to look at stigma and related experiences of parents/caregivers at different time-points in their child's life, or at pre- and post-engagement in a stigma reduction program.

Future studies should continue to examine how stigma effects this population of parents/caregivers. These findings also spark important clinical implications. Targeting the specific variables found to be relevant to this population has the potential to aid parents/caregivers in making more informed decisions, help parents/caregivers understand and cope with the emotional (e.g., depression) and behavioral (e.g., help-seeking) aspects of stigma they may face, as well as generally improve efficacy of anti-stigma interventions. For instance, Corrigan and colleagues (2014) identified and ranked important aspects of anti-stigma programs. Targeting a specific population, presenters identifying as a person with lived experience, including stories from people with lived experience, and discussing follow-up actions/targets have been identified as key features of anti-stigma programs. The current investigation provides support for specific anti-stigma programs for parents/caregivers of children with mental health challenges, for presenters to share lived experiences with depression and addressing barriers related to help-seeking, and for follow-up actions/targets to include addressing parent/caregiver depression symptoms and encouraging relevant help-seeking behaviors.

Selecting appropriate tools to adequately measure variables in a population of interest can be challenging. There is a need for measures specifically tailored to parents/caregivers of children with mental health challenges. A novel measure of vicarious stigma was utilized in this study, and adaptations were made to other existing measures in attempts to examine this population. Future community-based participatory research should investigate the content validity of adapting existing measures or creating new measures to better examine this population. Further research studying the psychometric properties of The Vicarious Stigma Scale as well as exploring the construct of vicarious stigma more broadly should also be considered. It is necessary to more comprehensively investigate vicarious stigma, and have good measures of this construct, to more fully understand and investigate the stigma experiences of parents/caregivers of children with mental health challenges.

5.3   Conclusions

This study adds to the literature examining the stigma experienced by parents/caregivers of children with mental health challenges, and continues the further investigation of a measure for the construct of vicarious stigma. Results suggest overlap in parents'/caregivers' emotional experiences of public stigma, self-stigma, and vicarious stigma as associated with higher levels of depression symptoms and differentially associated with help-seeking. Additional research is needed to better understand the many aspects related to stigma experienced by parents/caregivers of children with mental health challenges. Future research should include a more diverse sample regarding parent/caregiver and child characteristics. This line of inquiry has the potential to inform targeted anti-stigma interventions to ensure better outcomes for not only parents/caregivers, but also their children with mental health challenges.